Coronary Artery Disease

Causes, Symptoms and Treatments

Coronary Artery Disease

Causes, Symptoms and Treatments

Published by iConcept Press

Coronary Artery Disease – Causes, Symptoms and Treatments

Publisher: iConcept Press Ltd.

ISBN: 978-1-922227-92-8

Printed in the United States of America

𝄢Concept
Press Ltd.

www.iconceptpress.com

Contents

Preface

Coronary artery disease, or more commonly known as heart disease, is usually a result of plaque buildup in coronary arteries, a condition called atherosclerosis. This book covers original research with a clinical emphasis as well as advances in laboratory research that contribute to the understanding of coronary artery disease about its causes, symptoms and treatments. There are totally 6 chapters in this book. Chapter 1 proposes a basis for the establishment of effective rehabilitation planning. It discusses the clinical effect of 8-week rehabilitation program on physical, cognitive, and depressive symptoms and the variables influencing changes in depressive symptoms for the reduction of the psychological stress of chronic stroke. Chapter 2 provides an overview of our current understanding of cyclic nucleotide-driven protein kinase signals as essential components in arterial smooth muscle physiology and pathology underlying coronary artery disease. Chapter 3 discusses the presence of rhabdomyolysis as an adverse event after concomitant use of statins and antimicrobial agents and mechanisms involved to these interactions.

Chapter 4 aims to provide the extended version of presently published content on chitosan activities towards platelet and blood coagulation mechanisms. Since we are exploring on platelet activities which involve in the coagulation process, as a new contribution to the society, chitosan-based hemostatic agents could be a new strategy biomaterial to achieve hemostasis. Chapter 5 highlights the major findings and recent advances in the study of micro-biota-dependent mechanism involved in the development of Coronary Artery Disease (CAD) and discuss important roles of probiotic bacteria and plant compounds in prevention and treatment of CAD. Chapter 6 discusses the value of heart rate in the physiopathology and management of coronary artery disease. Physiology of heart rate value is discussed, along with topics that relate heart rate to endothelial dysfunction, atherosclerosis, hypertension, and other co-morbidities that predispose to coronary artery disease. The role of inflammation and autonomic nervous system are also presented.

Editing and publishing a book is never an easy task. Each chapter in this book has gone through a peer review, a selection and an editing process so as to guarantee its quality. Without the supports and contributions of the authors and reviewers, this book can never be able to complete. We would like to thank all of the authors in this book and all of the reviewers who participated in the reviewing process: Maria Jesus Casuso-Holgado,

Antonella Cecchettini, Leanne L. Cribbs, Jagadeesha K. Dammanahalli, Desiderio Favarato, Deanna L. Gibson, Maryam Goudarzi, Michiel B Haeseker, Paul J. Higgins, Xu Hu, Takeshi Ikeda, Shengyang Jiang, Takako Kaneko-Kawano, Maria Teresa La Rovere, O. J. T. McCarty, Virginia M Miller, Grace M Moran, Franco Morelli, David Pérez-Cruzado, Nicolás R Robles, Ashish Kumar Sharma, Mika P. Tarvainen, Srinivasan N. Tirupati, P. O. Ughachukwu, Christos Voucharas, Tao Wang, Joyce Y. Wong and Mihkel Zilmer. We hope that you, the reader, will find this book interesting and useful. Any advices please feel free and are always welcome to tell us.

iConcept Press Editorial Office
July 2016

Chapter 1

The Importance of Cognitive and Physical Functions on Improvement in Depression of Patients with Chronic Stroke

Yeon-Gyu Jeong[1], Yeon-Jae Jeong[2], In-Hyuk Lim[3], Hyun-Sook Kim[3]

1 Introduction

Physical disability occurring from stroke was obliged for a great responsibility socially and domestically (Yoon, 2009). Most of the time, stroke occurs during senior years which brings a big change in ones social activity and independency that leads to a decrease in ones physical ability (Yoon, 2009). If the subjects with stroke do not receive a proper protection and support physically, psychologically, and socially, it may result in an emotional pain such as mental regression, depression, discouragement, and anxiety (Rhee *et al.*, 1988). These mental disorders of chronic stroke continue for a long period throughout one's life and affects a lot on his/her quality of life (Lawrence & Christie, 1979). Nevertheless, stroke patients' social and psychological issues are underestimated among the medical society. Therefore, psychological treatment should be held with the physical treatment in order to improve the patient's quality of life. Since 20 years ago, Korea had a great interest in post-stroke depression and has been coming up with variety of results on the relationship between the time stroke occurs and the effects of it (Sharpe *et al.*, 1990; Wilkinson *et al.*, 1997). However, the research on the change in depression still lacks in its quality and quantity. Clinicians who treats stroke also acknowledge about the post-stroke depression but they are most likely to treat them as a simple physical/psychological symptom which can be taken care with less interest or

[1] Department of Physical Therapy, Sangji University, Republic of Korea
[2] Rehabilitation Medicine, Hanyang University Medical Center, Republic of Korea
[3] Department of Physical Therapy, Yeoju Institute of Technology, Republic of Korea

even be ignored. Accordingly, the main purpose of this study is to analyze the clinical effect of 8-week rehabilitation program on physical, cognitive, and depressive symptoms; secondly to explore the changes in cognitive, physical, and depressive symptoms after 8 weeks rehabilitation by groups with and without depressive symptoms; and finally to investigate other variables influencing changes in depressive symptoms for the reduction of the psychological stress of chronic stroke in order to propose a basis for the establishment of effective rehabilitation planning.

2   Subjects and Methods

This cross-sectional study conducted with 120 subjects, diagnosed with stroke, who were undergoing the rehabilitation for physical, occupational, and cognitive therapy (each 30 minutes, 5 times a week, 8 weeks) at a university hospital rehabilitation center located in Gyeonggi-Do province, from January 2008 to December 2009. Any subjects who had a history of mental disorders such as dementia, depression prior to stroke, anxiety disorders, having anti-depression medications, and difficulties in communication were excluded from the research. The present study was supported by Catholic University and approved by Catholic University Institutional Review Boards (Approval # CUMC10U026), and all of data were collected anonymously by the electronic medical record.

Based on the 8 weeks of rehabilitation, we collected the general characteristics such as the sex, age, marital status, caregiver, type of insurance, and decision-maker, health-related characteristics such as smoke, drink alcohol, diabetes, hypertension, cardiac disorder, hyperlipidemia, and history of pre-stroke, and disease-related characteristics such as lesion region, lesion type, duration of the onset of stroke, and whether the patient has a depression currently with clinical findings measured before and after treatment of physical, functional, and cognitive function, respectively, on every subject with chronic stroke.

The "Beck Depression Inventory" (BDI) was developed by Beck (Beck *et al.*, 1961), which is a survey method used commonly to evaluate the depression. It has 21 questions, each of which are answered on a 4-point scale with a higher score signifying greater depression symptoms. In this study it was used as the measurement for measuring the depression levels of subjects with chronic stroke. Also, it was classified by cutoff point of 21 scores, because it corresponds to cultural norms regarding depression in South Korea (Hahn *et al.*, 1986). The intrarater reliability has an intraclass correlation coefficient (ICC) of 0.94 (Hahn *et al.*, 1986).

A measuring tool for cognitive impairment was used by "Mini-Mental State Examination" (MMSE), which is also known to find cognitive impairment within the patients with a serious dementia as well (Folstein *et al.*, 1975). In this study, we used Mini-Mental State Examination-Korean (MMSE-K) to correspond to Korean reality, resulting in a tool consisting of 30 questions (Park & Kwon, 1989). The intrarater reliability of reliability is 0.99 (Park *et al.*, 2000).

The "Modified Bathel Index" (MBI) was developed by Shah (Shah *et al.*, 1989), which is known to be a sensitive rating scale which is a modified version of the original Bathel Index (Mahoney & Barthel, 1965). In this study it was used as the measurement for measuring ADLs of subjects with chronic stroke. We used the "Korean Modified Bathel Index" (K-MBI) to correspond to Korean reality, resulting in a tool consisting of 10 questions. The intrarater and interrater of reliability are 0.89, 0.95 (Son *et al.*, 2010). All the results were divided into 2 categories with better groups counted as > 25% improvement, and the others as less-improvement by 8-week rehabilitation.

The characteristics of the subjects are presented as frequencies and percentages using descriptive statistics. A *t*-test or analysis of variance (ANOVA) for categorical independent variables was conducted in order to examine the differences in changes of depressive symptoms through rehabilitation between groups attending to general, health-related, disease-related, and functioning-related characteristics. Additionally, we examined the changes in cognitive, physical, and depressive symptoms after 8 weeks rehabilitation program by groups without and with depressive symptoms, classified by cutoff point 21 scores using paired *t*-test or independent *t*-test. Finally, significant variables ($p < 0.05$) in the univariate analyses were entered into the hierarchical multiple regression analyses to identify predictors of improvement or worsening of depression through 8-week rehabilitation. These predictors were then tested for multicollinearity to prevent over-parameterization of the prediction model. The general and health-related characteristics of the stroke patients were entered in the first step and disease-related characteristics were entered in the second step, using the mode of one at a time and blocks. Each of the function-related variables of whether subjects with chronic stroke had depression, have improvement of ADLs, and cognitive functions more than before by rehabilitation, were successively entered in the prediction model using stepwise mode. The significance level was set at 0.05 (2-sided). Statistical analysis was performed utilizing SPSS ver. 17.0.

3   Results

As shown in Table 1, the relationship between all domains of characteristics of stroke and the change in depression resulted in significantly positive associa tion with having had a cardiac disorder ($t = 3.76$, $p < 0.05$) and depression symptoms ($t = 25.51$, $p < 0.001$), while the relationship with lesion on left brain($t = 2.94$, $p < 0.05$), was negative. Also, the relationship between the change in depression and clinical findings by 8-week rehabilitation was significantly positive with improved ADLs ($t = 2.10$, $p < 0.05$) and cognitive functions ($t = 2.48$, $p < 0.05$).

Furthermore, the results of changes in BDI, MMSE-K, and MBI scores after 8 weeks of rehabilitation by groups without and with depression symptoms are shown in Table 2. The group with depressive symptoms was significant higher on depressive scores, measured by BDI before ($t = -15.16$, $p < 0.01$) and after ($t = -6.00$, $p < 0.01$) 8 weeks of rehabilitation than group without depressive symptoms. However, the group with depressive symptoms was significantly improved with 8-week rehabilitation program (t

		Factors	N(%)	The changes of depressive symptoms		
				Mean ± SD	T / F	p
General characteristics	Gender	Male	72(60.0)	−1.42 ± 7.18	0.20	0.66
		Female	48(40.0)	−2.04 ± 7.93		
	Age	< 40	15(12.5)	−0.20 ± 7.66	0.34	0.71
		40 ~ < 64	44(36.7)	−1.73 ± 7.52		
		≥ 64	61(50.8)	−1.98 ± 7.45		
	Marital status	Unmarried	13(10.8)	−1.79 ± 7.47	0.29	0.59
		Married or co–habiting	107(89.2)	−0.62 ± 7.61		
	Caregivers	Self	3(2.5)	−6.67 ± 10.07	1.56	0.22
		Family	57(47.5)	−0.61 ± 6.54		
		Others (public or private facility)	60(50.0)	−2.42 ± 8.08		
	Decision maker	Family	103(85.8)	−1.80 ± 7.23	0.22	0.64
		Self	17(14.2)	−0.88 ± 8.93		
	Insurance	Health	98(81.7)	−2.22 ± 7.44	2.36	0.08
		Automobile	7(5.8)	2.43 ± 6.27		
		Industrial disaster	7(5.8)	3.86 ± 7.01		
		Others (1,2 type Medical aids)	8(6.7)	−3.25 ± 6.98		
Health-related characteristics	Smoking	Yes	46(38.3)	−1.07 ± 7.06	0.48	0.49
		No	74(61.7)	−2.04 ± 7.73		
	Drinking	Yes	50(41.7)	−1.20 ± 7.71	0.33	0.57
		No	70(58.3)	−2.00 ± 7.74		
	Hyper-tension	Yes	80(66.7)	−1.78 ± 7.74	0.05	0.82
		No	40(33.3)	−1.45 ± 6.96		
	Hyper-lipidemia	Yes	27(22.5)	−0.89 ± 7.08	0.38	0.54
		No	93(77.5)	−1.89 ± 7.59		
	Heart disease	Yes	12(10.0)	−5.58 ± 6.69	3.76	0.04
		No	108(90.0)	−1.23 ± 7.44		
	Pre-stroke history	Yes	17(14.2)	−3.00 ± 5.55	0.63	0.43
		No	103(55.5)	−1.45 ± 7.73		

Continued on next page...

...Continued from previous page

Disease-related characteristics	Duration after onset (month)	< 3	78(65.1)	−2.49 ± 7.71	2.16	0.10
		3 ~ < 6	16(13.3)	1.00 ± 6.47		
		6 ~ < 12	13(10.8)	1.69 ± 7.84		
		≥ 12	13(10.8)	−3.38 ± 5.32		
	Stroke type	Infarction	61(50.8)	−2.08 ± 7.53	0.25	0.78
		Hemorrhage	57(47.5)	−1.18 ± 7.55		
		Both	2(1.7)	−3.00 ± 1.41		
	Side of lesion	Left hemisphere	37(30.8)	1.11 ± 6.64	2.94	0.04
		Right hemisphere	63(52.5)	−3.30 ± 7.65		
		Both	17(14.2)	−1.29 ± 6.52		
		Brainstem & others	3(2.5)	−3.67 ± 11.5		
Function-related characteristics	Depression	Yes (> 21 scores)	27(22.5)	−7.31 ± 7.11	25.51	< 0.001
		No (≤ 21 scores)	93(77.5)	−0.01 ± 6.76		
	ADLs function[4]	High (≥ 25% improvement)	50(41.7)	−3.40 ± 7.88	2.1	0.038
		Low (< 25% improvement)	70(58.3)	−0.51 ± 6.99		
	Cognitive function	High (≥ 25% improvement)	46(38.3)	−6.21 ± 6.44	2.48	0.015
		Low (< 25% improvement)	74(61.7)	−1.07 ± 7.41		

Table 1: The relationships between general, health, disease, and function-related characteristics and changes of depressive symptoms after 8 weeks of rehabilitation in stroke patients.

---

[4] ADLs, activities of daily living

		Group without depressive symptoms (N = 93)	Group with depressive symptoms (N = 27)	t^5	p
BDI, Mean±SD	Pre	8.85 ± 5.09	26.41 ± 5.98	−15.15	0.00
	Post	8.87 ± 7.39	18.93 ± 8.55	−6.00	0.00
	t^6	−0.03	5.53		
	P	0.98	0.00		
MMSE[7], Mean±SD	Pre	24.45 ± 3.83	21.89 ± 3.84	3.06	0.00
	Post	25.38 ± 3.42	24.59 ± 2.85	0.25	0.17
	t^2	−3.61	−4.01		
	P	0.00	0.00		
MBI[8], Mean±SD	Pre	57.34 ± 27.16	43.44 ± 25.40	2.37	0.02
	Post	69.41 ± 26.01	65.07 ± 26.31	0.76	0.45
	t^2	−9.15	−6.33		
	p	0.00	0.00		

Table 2: Changes in cognitive, physical, and depressive symptoms after 8 weeks rehabilitation program by groups without and with depressive symptoms.

=5.53, $p < 0.01$). Although group with depressive symptoms was significantly lower on cognitive status ($t = -3.01$, $p < 0.01$) and ADLs ($t = 2.37$, $p < 0.05$) at the initial evaluation than group without depressive symptoms, both groups showed improvement in cognitive status ($t = -3.61$, $p < 0.01$/ $t = -4.01$, $p < 0.01$, respectively) and ADLs ($t = -9.15$, $p < 0.01$/ $t = -6.33$, $p < 0.01$, respectively) with 8-week rehabilitation program irrespective of depression.

The results of hierarchical multiple regression analyses are presented in Table 3. As a result of analyzing factors influencing the change in depression symptom of chronic stroke by rehabilitation, as well as modifying the efficacy of other variables in the final step, the overall model, the subjects with having had the cardiac disorder ($\beta = -4.98$, $p < 0.05$) and depression ($\beta = -6.37$, $p < 0.05$), improved ADLs ($\beta = -3.59$, $p < 0.05$), and cognitive functions ($\beta = -4.21$, $p < 0.05$) were identified as significant predictors of improvement of depression.

---

[5] comparison of cognitive and functional recovery within groups
[6] comparison of cognitive and functional recovery between groups
[7] MMSE, mini-mental state of examination
[8] MBI, modified barthel index

	Factors	Categories	Model 1[9] β	Model 2 β	Model 3 β	Model 4 β	Model 5 β
General characteristics	Sex	Male	Ref.	Ref.	Ref.	Ref.	Ref.
		Female	−0.28	0.57	0.62	0.16	0.25
	Age	< 40	0.31	0.43	1.38	0.95	0.89
		40 ~ 64	Ref.	Ref.	Ref.	Ref.	Ref.
		≥ 64	0.09	0.60	1.42	1.29	1.30
	Insurance	Health	Ref.	Ref.	Ref.	Ref.	Ref.
		Auto-mobile	4.50	3.04	5.45	4.96	4.50
		Industrial dis-aster	5.60	7.70	7.16	6.66	6.66
		Medical aids	−0.98	2.17	2.31	2.13	2.28
Health-related characteristics	Cardiac disorder	Yes	Ref.	Ref.	Ref.	Ref.	Ref.
		No	3.81	3.63*	5.26*	5.50*	5.39*
	Pre-stroke history	Yes	Ref.	Ref.	Ref.	Ref.	Ref.
		No	0.22	0.14	−0.70	−0.65	−0.82
Disease-related characteristics	Duration after onset stroke (month)	< 3		Ref.	Ref.	Ref.	Ref.
		3 ~ < 6		1.90	0.27	0.26	0.16
		6 ~ < 12		5.04	3.42	3.16	3.07
		≥ 12		−1.38	−0.46	−0.71	−1.14
	Stroke lesion	Left hemisphere		Ref.	Ref.	Ref.	Ref.
		Right hemisphere		−4.00*	−2.13	−2.22	−2.31
		Both		−5.11*	−5.11*	−5.05*	−4.98*
		Brainstem & Other		−8.31	−6.41	−5.62	−5.44

Continued on next page...

[9] *$p < 0.05$

...Continued from previous page

					Ref.	Ref.	Ref.
Function-related characteristics	Depression	No (≤ 21 scores)			Ref.	Ref.	Ref.
		Yes (> 21 scores)			–7.15*	–6.60*	–6.37*
	ADLs function[10]	Low				Ref.	Ref.
		High				–3.75*	–3.59*
	Cognitive function	Low					Ref.
		High					–4.21*
R^2			0.08	0.19	0.32	0.38	0.48
R^2 Change				0.11	0.13	0.07	0.10
F				1.78	3.22	3.16	2.98

Table 3: Hierarchical multiple regression with the changes in depression symptoms after 8 weeks of rehabilitation.

4   Discussion

Every investigation on the frequency of post-stroke depression seemed to have a small amount of difference but it is reported to be in a 20~60% range in average (Paolucci, 2008). In present study, the frequency of post-stroke depression had the result of 22.5% which was lower than 30% of other studies (House *et al.*, 1990; Paolucci, 2008). That's why we have got the cutoff points of 21 when all the other studies had 10 points.

Post-stroke depression occasionally happens in the acute as well as the chronic stages that have occurred following 2~3 years (Robinson & Price, 1982). Post-stroke depression increases the amount of damage neurologically and psychologically which ends up in a bigger damage in ADLs. Since these symptoms increase the suicide rate as well as the death rate which relates as a disturbance factor of rehabilitation, depression should be treated with more care and interest in post-stroke treatments (Carod-Artal *et al.*, 2009). Due to these mentioned above, this research elicited the preventive factors that cause changes in depressive symptoms among stroke patients by 8-week rehabilitation and compared how much the related factors affected in change in depression. In these 8 weeks of rehabilitation, there resulted in five main variables of whether the patients previously had a cardiac disorder, left lesion of brain, depression, and better activities of daily living and cognitive function by treatment. With all these variables they showed the 48.3% of the total change.

First of all, the general, health-related (cardiac disorder, $\beta = -5.26$, $p < 0.05$), and disease-related characteristics (left hemisphere, $\beta = 5.11$, $p < 0.05$), depression ($\beta = -7.15$, $p < 0.05$) explained 32% of the variance in changes in depressive symptoms, of which the variable that had the most influence on the change in depression by rehabilitation was

---

[10] ADLs, activities of daily living

whether the patient had depression in the beginning of the treatment (12.5%). According to the research of the senior depressive patients, regular exercise or leisure activities ($r = 0.16$–0.26, $p < 0.05$) reduced depression, which increased the life satisfaction after all (Kwon & Kim, 2008; McAuley et al., 1995). Even though it did not match with participants of present study, the benefit of exercises for decreasing depression was identical in context, with the present study. However, other research didn't show significant results of depression symptoms by the physical therapy itself even though their depression scores (mean difference: -0.17) reduced by a little (Yi & Jeong, 2001), which was in contrast to our significant study results (mean difference: -7.48). It is likely that our study focused on a broad spectrum of rehabilitation, i.e., physical, function performance on ADLs, and cognitive exercises compared with only physical exercises of previous study (Yi & Jeong, 2001).

Second, the general, health-related (cardiac disorder, $\beta = -5.39$, $p < 0.05$), and disease-related characteristics (left hemisphere, $\beta = 4.98$, $p < 0.05$), depression ($\beta = -6.37$, $p < 0.05$), ADLs ($\beta = -3.59$, $p < 0.05$), and cognition ($\beta = -4.21$, $p < 0.05$) explained 48% of the variance in changes in depressive symptoms, of which the improvement of cognitive function had the influence on the change in depression (10.1%) even though lot of studies showed that there are not any correlation between depression and cognitive function (Lipsey et al., 1984; Robinson et al., 2000). Andersen (Andersen et al., 1996) claimed that disorder in cognitive function was the main reason of depression among stroke patients since the patients who showed an improvement in cognitive function showed an improvement in depression. Also, the stroke patients who have an improvement in cognitive function (mean difference: 4.1) in the next 3 months of the onset of stroke showed a great improvement for their depression (Murata et al., 2000), which was same as our study results (mean difference: 4.0). Therefore, it implies that the cognitive function has to be taken care of first in order to improve the depression.

Third, the general, health-related (cardiac disorder, $\beta = -5.50$, $p < 0.05$), and disease-related characteristics (left hemisphere, $\beta = 5.05$, $p < 0.05$), depression ($\beta = -6.60$, $p < 0.05$), and ADLs ($\beta = -3.75$, $p < 0.05$) explained 38% of the variance in changes in depressive symptoms, of which the improvement of ADLs had influence on the change in depression (6.5%).

According to Robinson (Robinson et al., Starr, 1984) and Snaphan (Snaphaan et al., 2009), the stoke patients who had an improvement on his/her of ADLs showed an improvement in depression ($r = 0.39$), which was same as our study results ($r = 0.19$). Other studies showed that depression and ADLs had a correlation since the stroke patients who had depression were more dependent on themselves' activity with heavier psychological disorders than those who did not have depression (Morris et al., 1992; Robinson, 2003). However, other studies found no significant relationship between functional disability and post-stroke depression (Gillen et al., 2001; Nannetti et al., 2005; van de Weg et al., 1999). In Korea where there is inadequate social insurance, the prolonged hospitalization required in stroke with subsequent inability for returning to work due to functional impairment is a great economic burden on the family. This further contributes to functional impairment, a potential great risk factor of post-stroke depression in Korea (Aben et al., 2003; Jeong et al., 2015).

Last of all, the general, health-related (cardiac disorder, $\beta = -3.63$, $p < 0.05$), and disease-related characteristics (left hemisphere, $\beta = 5.11$, $p < 0.05$) explained 19% of the variance in changes in depressive symptoms, of which the left brain lesion and cardiac disorder had influence on the change in depression (11.1%). There is still controversial on relationship between stroke lesion and post-stroke depression. In a systemic review by Carson (Carson et al., 2000), 38 studies found no significant difference between side of lesion and post-stroke depression, 7 reported increased risk with right lesions, and 2 reported increased risk with left lesioin (Carson et al., 2000). However, in present study, subjects with depressive symptoms were more likely to have left lesion of stroke lesion, which was same as other studies (Verdelho et al., 2004). When compared with previous studies, there may be varying relationship between side of lesion and post-stroke depression just as Carson (Carson et al., 2000). And, in the present study, patients with cardiac disorder had a higher possibility of having a severe depression compared to the patients who did not. The result was supported by other studies, that patients with myocardial infarction and coronary disease had a higher rate of getting depression (Carney et al., 1987; Thomas et al., 2003). However, Leentjens (Leentjens et al., 2006) stated that there were not any correlation between hypertension, diabetes, cardiac disorder, smoking, and etc with depression.

Additionally, we distinguished the group with depression from the group without depression with a cutoff score of 21 for the BDI to explore changes in cognitive, physical, and depressive symptoms after 8 weeks rehabilitation program. Although groups with and without depressive symptoms did not result in subject categories that accorded with the predetermined standards, we confirmed improvement in cognitive status and ADLs with 8 weeks of rehabilitation irrespective of depression. The previous study (Chemerinski et al., 2001) reported that stroke patients with either major or minor depression symptoms at the initial evaluation showed the same amount of ADLs recovery, which was the same with our study results. Other studies also found that improved cognitive function and functional independence had a protective effect on post-stroke depression (Robinson et al., 2000; Snaphaan et al., 2009). Considering cognitive and ADLs recovery as predictors of improvement in depressive symptoms mentioned above, post-stroke depression, rehabilitation for the post-stroke depression should be focused on improvement in cognition and ADLs independent of presence of depression.

The limitations of this study are as follows. First, because our sampling consisted of limited patients on a single university hospital and was lack of a control group who did not receive intervention, the current findings cannot be generalized to all people with stroke. Second, this study ruled out aphasia patients with stroke, since aphasia could have been caused by left brain lesion which could affect our results. We need to include the aphasia patients in further study. Also, because the present study was conducted for short period of 8-week rehabilitation, generalization of these results was inconclusive unless further studies on long-term of rehabilitation on the change in depression symptoms are performed. Finally, we did not consider the variables such as financial problem, social support, self-efficacy, and self-esteem. According to Aben (Aben et al., 2002), depression patients with stroke have a great influence on psychological and environmental parts. However, the present study has meaningful results to suggest that post-stroke depression was mediated by improved cognitive and functional ability, which could be treated with rehabilitation irrespective of depression. In addition, these results also provide objective data on studies which have few on the relationship of depression and rehabilitation. To clarify the effectiveness on which specific domains of rehabilitation are appropriate for reducing post-stroke depression, further study considering these limitations is needed

5   Conclusion

The post-stroke depression should be focused on improvement in cognition and ADLs through rehabilitation independent of presence of depression. Also, the clinicians should comprehend and share the psychological and physical affliction, developing back-up programs, and making them comprehensively available to support the psychological and physical health of subjects with chronic stroke.

Acknowledgments

We want to thank all the patients, interviewers, and all the facilities of the general hospitals and private rehabilitation centers that participated in this study. The authors wish to express their gratitude to all of them.

References

Aben, I., Denollet, J., Lousberg, R., Verhey, F., Wojciechowski, F., & Honig, A. (2002). *Personality and vulnerability to depression in stroke patients: a 1-year prospective follow-up study. Stroke, 33(10), 2391–2395.*

Aben, I., Verhey, F., Strik, J., Lousberg, R., Lodder, J., & Honig, A. (2003). *A comparative study into the one year cumulative incidence of depression after stroke and myocardial infarction. J Neurol Neurosurg Psychiatry, 74(5), 581–585.*

Andersen, G., Vestergaard, K., Riis, J. O., & Ingeman-Nielsen, M. (1996). *Dementia of depression or depression of dementia in stroke? Acta Psychiatr Scand, 94(4), 272–278.*

Beck, A. T., Ward, C. H., Mendelson, M., Mock, J., & Erbaugh, J. (1961). *An inventory for measuring depression. Arch Gen Psychiatry, 4, 561–571.*

Carney, R. M., Rich, M. W., Tevelde, A., Saini, J., Clark, K., & Jaffe, A. S. (1987). *Major depressive disorder in coronary artery disease. Am J Cardiol, 60(16), 1273–1275.*

Carod-Artal, F. J., Ferreira Coral, L., Trizotto, D. S., & Menezes Moreira, C. (2009). *Poststroke depression: prevalence and determinants in Brazilian stroke patients. Cerebrovasc Dis, 28(2), 157–165.*

Carson, A. J., MacHale, S., Allen, K., Lawrie, S. M., Dennis, M., House, A., & Sharpe, M. (2000). Depression after stroke and lesion location: a systematic review. Lancet, 356(9224), 122–126.

Chemerinski, E., Robinson, R. G., & Kosier, J. T. (2001). Improved recovery in activities of daily living associated with remission of poststroke depression. Stroke, 32(1), 113–117.

Folstein, M. F., Folstein, S. E., & McHugh, P. R. (1975). "Mini-mental state". A practical method for grading the cognitive state of patients for the clinician. J Psychiatr Res, 12(3), 189–198.

Gillen, R., Tennen, H., McKee, T. E., Gernert-Dott, P., & Affleck, G. (2001). Depressive symptoms and history of depression predict rehabilitation efficiency in stroke patients. Arch Phys Med Rehabil, 82(12), 1645–1649.

Hahn, H. M., Yum, T. H., Shin, Y. W., Kim, K. H., Yoon, D. J., & Chung, K. J. (1986). A standardization study of beck depression inventory in Korea. J Korean Neuropsychiatr Assoc, 25(3), 487–500.

House, A., Dennis, M., Warlow, C., Hawton, K., & Molyneux, A. (1990). Mood disorders after stroke and their relation to lesion location. A CT scan study. Brain, 113 (Pt 4), 1113–1129.

Jeong, Y. G., Myong, J. P., & Koo, J. W. (2015). The modifying role of caregiver burden on predictors of quality of life of caregivers of hospitalized chronic stroke patients. Disabil Health J, 8(4), 619–625.

Kwon, W. A., & Kim, H. S. (2008). A study on the correlation between the types of leisure activity and depression in the elderly. J Kor Soc Phys The, 20(4), 51–59.

Lawrence, L., & Christie, D. (1979). Quality of life after stroke: a three-year follow-up. Age Ageing, 8(3), 167–172.

Leentjens, A. F., Aben, I., Lodder, J., & Verhey, F. R. (2006). General and disease-specific risk factors for depression after ischemic stroke: a two-step Cox regression analysis. Int Psychogeriatr, 18(4), 739–748.

Lipsey, J. R., Robinson, R. G., Pearlson, G. D., Rao, K., & Price, T. R. (1984). Nortriptyline treatment of post-stroke depression: a double-blind study. Lancet, 1(8372), 297–300.

Mahoney, F. I., & Barthel, D. W. (1965). FUNCTIONAL EVALUATION: THE BARTHEL INDEX. Md State Med J, 14, 61–65.

McAuley, E., Shaffer, S. M., & Rudolph, D. (1995). Affective responses to acute exercise in elderly impaired males: the moderating effects of self-efficacy and age. Int J Aging Hum Dev, 41(1), 13–27.

Morris, P. L., Raphael, B., & Robinson, R. G. (1992). Clinical depression is associated with impaired recovery from stroke. Med J Aust, 157(4), 239–242.

Murata, Y., Kimura, M., & Robinson, R. G. (2000). Does cognitive impairment cause post-stroke depression? Am J Geriatr Psychiatry, 8(4), 310–317.

Nannetti, L., Paci, M., Pasquini, J., Lombardi, B., & Taiti, P. G. (2005). Motor and functional recovery in patients with post-stroke depression. Disabil Rehabil, 27(4), 170–175.

Paolucci, S. (2008). Epidemiology and treatment of post-stroke depression. Neuropsychiatr Dis Treat, 4(1), 145–154.

Park, J. H., & Kwon, Y. C. (1989). Standardization of Korean version of the mini-mental state examination (MMSE-K) for use in the elderly: PartII. diagnostic validity. J Korean Neuropsychiatr Assoc, 28(3), 508–513.

Park, R. J., Lee, H. O., Kim, S. H. (2000). Correlation analysis between MBI and MMSE after exercise program for dementia elderly. J Kor Soc Phys Ther, 12(2), 83–93.

Rhee, I. G., Han, H. Y., Kim, H. S., Nah, Y. S., & Ahn, K. H. (1988). Emotional disorder of stroke patients. J Korean Acad Rehab Med, 12(1), 33–38.

Robinson, R. G. (2003). Poststroke depression: prevalence, diagnosis, treatment, and disease progression. Biol Psychiatry, 54(3), 376–387.

Robinson, R. G., & Price, T. R. (1982). Post-stroke depressive disorders: a follow-up study of 103 patients. Stroke, 13(5), 635–641.

Robinson, R. G., Schultz, S. K., Castillo, C., Kopel, T., Kosier, J. T., Newman, R. M., . . . Starkstein, S. E. (2000). Nortriptyline versus fluoxetine in the treatment of depression and in short-term recovery after stroke: a placebo-controlled, double-blind study. Am J Psychiatry, 157(3), 351–359.

Robinson, R. G., Starr, L. B., Lipsey, J. R., Rao, K., & Price, T. R. (1984). A two-year longitudinal study of post-stroke mood disorders: dynamic changes in associated variables over the first six months of follow-up. Stroke, 15(3), 510–517.

Shah, S., Vanclay, F., & Cooper, B. (1989). Improving the sensitivity of the Barthel Index for stroke rehabilitation. J Clin Epidemiol, 42(8), 703–709.

Sharpe, M., Hawton, K., House, A., Molyneux, A., Sandercock, P., Bamford, J., & Warlow, C. (1990). Mood disorders in long-term survivors of stroke: associations with brain lesion location and volume. Psychol Med, 20(4), 815–828.

Snaphaan, L., van der Werf, S., Kanselaar, K., & de Leeuw, F. E. (2009). Post-stroke depressive symptoms are associated with post-stroke characteristics. Cerebrovasc Dis, 28(6), 551–557.

Son, H. H., Oh, J. L., & Park, R. J. (2010). The effect of an exercise program on activities of daily living (ADL), balance and cognition in elderly individuals with alzheimer's disease and vascular dementia. J Kor Phys Ther, 12(1), 53–60.

Thomas, A. J., O'Brien, J. T., Barber, R., McMeekin, W., & Perry, R. (2003). A neuropathological study of periventricular white matter hyperintensities in major depression. J Affect Disord, 76(1–3), 49–54.

van de Weg, F. B., Kuik, D. J., & Lankhorst, G. J. (1999). Post-stroke depression and functional outcome: a cohort study investigating the influence of depression on functional recovery from stroke. Clin Rehabil, 13(3), 268–272.

Verdelho, A., Henon, H., Lebert, F., Pasquier, F., & Leys, D. (2004). Depressive symptoms after stroke and relationship with dementia: A three-year follow-up study. Neurology, 62(6), 905–911.

Wilkinson, P. R., Wolfe, C. D., Warburton, F. G., Rudd, A. G., Howard, R. S., Ross-Russell, R. W., & Beech, R. R. (1997). A long-term follow-up of stroke patients. Stroke, 28(3), 507–512.

Yi, S. J., & Jeong, S. Y. (2001). Change of Depression According to Physical Therapy in Stroke Patients. J Kor Phys Ther, Journal, 13(1), 33–40.

Yoon, T. S. (2009). The influence of depressive symptoms on cognitive and functional recovery in chronic stroke patients. Masters Dissertation: Dong-guk University Graduate School of Medicine.

Chapter 2

Cyclic Nucleotide-driven Protein Kinase Signaling in Arterial Smooth Muscle (Patho)physiology

Andrew W. Holt[1], Lisandra E. de Castro Brás[1], David A. Tulis[1]

1 Introduction

Cardiovascular disease (CVD) constitutes the number one killer of individuals worldwide, accounting for nearly 30% of all deaths, and is considered a true global pandemic (World Health Organization, 2011). Of the many forms of CVD, coronary artery disease (CAD) is a primary contributor to and accounts for over half of all CVD-related deaths (American Heart Association (AHA), 2014; World Health Organization, 2011). Over many decades considerable basic science and clinical investigations have been performed aimed at identifying, characterizing and controlling the diverse and multifaceted mechanisms that underlie CAD and CVD; however, despite considerable progress outcomes from these studies have not been entirely effective and the number of individuals suffering and dying from these dreaded phenomena is still rising. In fact, in the United States alone it is estimated that the prevalence of CVD will increase 10% with greater than 40% of adults having some form of CVD in the next 20 years, coinciding with the economic burden of CVD that is expected to triple in that time frame (AHA, 2011). Undoubtedly, heightened efforts must be made on all fronts to combat the wide-ranging and complex mechanisms fundamental to CAD and CVD.

Numerous pathologic processes have been identified that serve as central foundations of CAD, and of these, coronary artery dysfunction and/or uncontrolled coronary artery growth are of major significance. In response to inimical stimuli as occurs during

[1] Department of Physiology, Brody School of Medicine, East Carolina University, Greenville, North Carolina, USA

pathogenesis of CAD and other vascular disorders, homeostatic and contractile arterial smooth muscle (ASM) undergoes phenotypic switching to become synthetic, migratory and proliferative (Thomas *et al.*, 1976; Ross, 1993, Davis *et al.*, 2006). This conversion of normally quiescent ASM into a growth-promoting embryonic phenotype is manifested as loss of contractile function and induction of a reorganized architecture complete with mural remodeling and neointima formation (Ross *et al.*, 1973; Liang *et al.*, 2014; Tulis, 2015). While this vascular remodeling initially serves as a compensatory adaptation it can progress into an uncontrolled, pathologic and self-perpetuating cascade with severe clinical repercussions. During the pathogenesis of atherosclerosis, a primary form of CAD, this process contributes significantly to the evolution of an emerging plaque and luminal obstruction concomitant with compromised blood flow. In the coronary circulation this pathology is of utmost concern as it elevates local vascular resistance and, in conjunction with extravascular systolic compression, can reduce local perfusion pressures and limit or eliminate local blood flow, resulting in focal ischemia and hypoxia or anoxia in downstream myocardium. Clearly, the impact of pathologic ASM growth and phenotypic modulation of ASM in CAD and other vascular disorders is highly critical and of utmost importance.

Many different biochemical, molecular, and cellular signaling processes have been identified and characterized as key regulators in the phenotypic switching of ASM cells and ensuing vessel wall remodeling. The multifaceted cyclic nucleotide pathways, comprised primarily of purine-based 3′,5′-cyclic adenosine monophosphate (cyclic AMP) and 3′,5′-cyclic guanosine monophosphate (cyclic GMP) and their downstream cascade of targets including diverse protein kinases, serve ubiquitous roles in normal vessel physiology and homeostasis but also in the pathogenesis of vascular dysfunction including CAD and associated occlusive disorders. Recent work from our lab and others has identified the serine (Ser)/threonine (Thr) kinases cyclic AMP-dependent protein kinase (PKA), cyclic GMP-dependent protein kinase (PKG), the calcium-activated phospholipid-dependent protein kinase C (PKC) and protein kinase D (PKD) as well as AMP-activated protein kinase (AMPK) as crucial controllers of ASM pathologic growth using a variety of experimental platforms and approaches. Using rodent primary and commercial ASM cells with pharmacologic, genetic, and molecular interventions we have documented capacity of these Ser/Thr kinases to control pathologic proliferation, migration and chemotaxis, matrix balance including the influence on matrix metalloproteinases (MMPs), apoptosis, and necrosis. We have observed the importance of Ser/Thr-specific protein phosphatases (PPs) in moderating kinase activities and in maintaining phosphorylative balance. Moreover, using whole animal models of injury-induced arterial growth we have verified biological ability of these pathways to operate in a whole body setting. Lastly, we have solidified many of these observations in rodent models by recapitulating them in human coronary ASM cells, thereby adding translational relevance to these intriguing basic science findings. Indeed, elucidation of the key influence of cyclic nucleotide-directed protein kinases on ASM anatomy and function provides important new perspectives on vessel wall biology and sheds light on potential novel targets that could be used to combat CAD and associated vascular occlusive disorders.

The purpose of this chapter is to highlight the importance of cyclic nucleotides and cyclic nucleotide-driven protein kinases in regulating ASM physiology and pathology in CAD. Discussion will cover fundamentals of arterial anatomy and physiology, an overview of CAD, and the influence of hemodynamics, fluid stresses, and matrix balance including roles for matrix-degrading MMPs. Thorough discussion is included for cyclic nucleotide signaling pathways including the emerging target of cyclic nucleotide-dependent Ser/Thr protein kinases, the cytoskeletal focal adhesion protein vasodilator-stimulated serum phosphoprotein (VASP), and a new family of pharmacologic agonists which have been gaining momentum as pivotal players in ASM growth regulation during CAD and CVD. This chapter will conclude with a short synopsis including some potential future directions for investigation that have appeal from both basic science and clinical perspectives.

2   Overview of Arterial Anatomy & Physiology

Before starting discussion of disease processes, a brief overview of basic anatomy and physiology of the arterial system is warranted. Within blood vessel walls there generally exist three concentric layers which may differ based on vessel size, anatomical location, and primary function (reviewed in Holt & Tulis, 2015). Starting from the blood-carrying lumen, the innermost blood vessel layer is termed the *tunica* (Latin for coat) *intima*, comprised of squamous arterial endothelial cells (AECs) sitting on an internal elastic lamina and a matrix protein-rich basement membrane. The *tunica intima* provides an important barrier between platelet-rich luminal blood and the highly thrombogenic sub-intimal layer. Intimal AECs also communicate with underlying medial wall ASM to regulate vascular tone and function; hence, this crucial intimal layer is largely responsible for controlling homeostatic blood vessel function. The *tunica intima* is also pivotal in the generation and liberation of autocrine, paracrine, and endocrine vasoactive factors that have capacity to modulate arterial physiology and pathobiology. The middle arterial layer is called the *tunica media* and is composed of spindle-shaped mononuclear ASM cells, sparse macrophages and fibroblasts, and an interstitial matrix. This muscular *tunica media* provides structural support to blood vessels and is the main functional tissue that controls vasoconstriction and vasodilation (and in turn, degree of blood flow) based on local tissue requirements. Adult medial ASM cells are normally fully differentiated and contractile, which enables their vasoreactivity and control of arterial tone and vascular resistance. These, in turn, direct distribution of blood flow in tissue-specific fashion based on local metabolic demands. Under homeostatic conditions, adult medial ASM cells are primarily quiescent, 'resting' in the non-proliferative G_0 phase of the cell cycle. In this differentiated state, ASM cells have low turnover and basal proliferative or synthetic activities and are dedicated to their primary function of constriction and relaxation. The outermost vascular layer is termed *tunica externa* or adventitia, which is separated from the medial wall by external elastic lamina and is composed of sparse ASM cells, nerve cells, fibroblasts, fat cells, and connective tissue that provide structural support as the extracellular matrix (ECM). In large conduit vessels the adventitia also contains its own blood supply or *vasa vasorum* that provides nutrients and oxygen to the thick muscular wall. A schematic of normal arterial wall anatomy containing an adventitia, medial wall, and intima is shown in Figure 1(a). In this diagram external and internal elastic laminae are also depicted. Figure 1(b) shows a photomicrograph of a high magnification cross-section from a sham-operated rat carotid artery including these essential layers and elastic laminae. Of note, disruption of the medial elastic laminae and basement membrane along with exaggerated focal intimal growth are shown (at asterisk) remnant from the sham surgery. Figure 1(c) shows a representative cross-section of an intact rat carotid artery with a thin intimal layer, a modest adventitia, and a completely patent lumen.

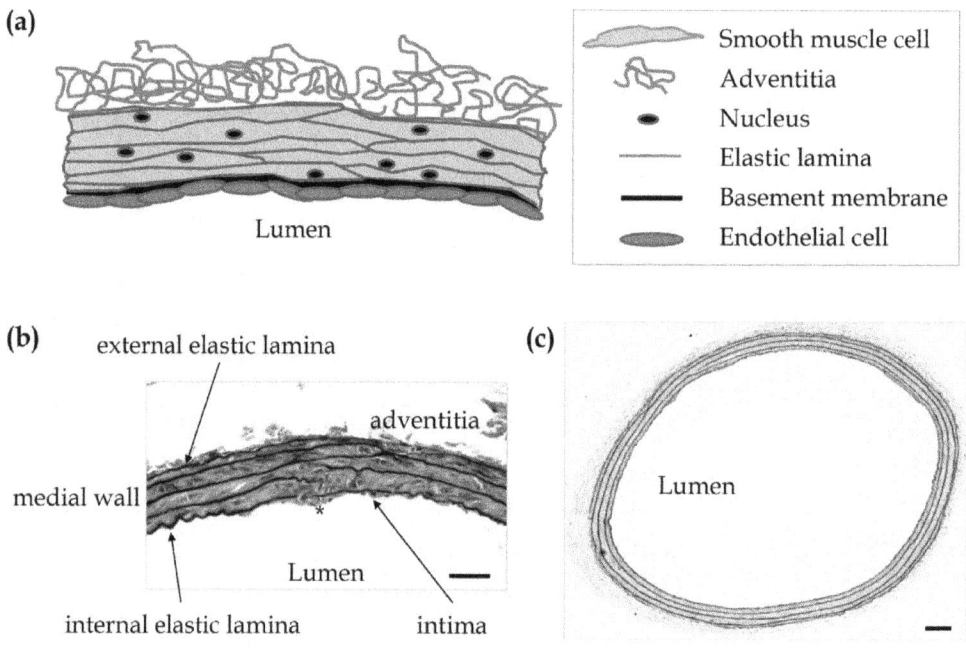

Figure 1: Arterial anatomy. **(a)** Schematic of normal arterial wall anatomy with corresponding legend. **(b)** Photomicrograph of a sham-operated Verhoeff/Van Giesen-stained cross-section of a rat artery showing adventitia, the external and internal elastic laminae, the medial wall and the intima. Remnants of the sham surgery are evident (at asterisk) as fractured laminae and focal intimal growth. Scale bar in B is 80 μm. **(c)** Photomicrograph of Verhoeff/Van Giesen-stained rat intact carotid artery cross-section with patent lumen and faint adventitial staining. Scale bar in C is 50 μm. Please refer to the online version for colored images for this figure.[2]

---

[2] https://www.iconceptpress.com/book/coronary-artery-disease--causes-symptoms-and-treatments/11000164/1411001255/

Physiologically, a major function of arteries is their ability to constrict and relax, in turn controlling vascular tone and resistance and blood flow to downstream tissues. Logically this is of critical importance in the provision of vital nutrients and oxygen to essential tissues and removal of metabolic by-products and carbon dioxide (CO_2). Blood vessels also operate as routes for the distribution of circulating hormones and other vasoactive factors as well as inflammatory mediators and platelets. Another function of blood vessels is their involvement in growth adaptations following exercise, in wound healing, or after surgical intervention. These normal vessel growth responses can involve arteriogenesis or adaptive and constructive vascular remodeling, angiogenesis (formation of new blood vessels from existing vessels), vasculogenesis (*de novo* formation of new blood vessels), arborization or branching of existing vessels, and/or collateralization to provide new blood supply to an existing vascular bed. Given the vital importance of these forms of homeostatic vessel growth, context must be considered when comparing normal versus pathologic ASM growth in the setting of CAD or CVD. Enlarged photomicrographs of human confluent coronary ASM cells showing morphology (top image) as well as G-actin (red) and F-actin (green) staining (bottom image) along with listings of characteristics of normal and pathologic ASM cells are shown in Figure 2.

3 Blood Flow & Hemodynamics

In our circulatory system there are four major types of blood flow: 1) pulsatile, 2) oscillatory, 3) laminar, and 4) turbulent (Davies *et al.*, 1992; Palumbo *et al.*, 2000). Pulsatile and oscillatory blood flows share common characteristics and result from periodic fluctuations in pulse waves corresponding to cardiac sinus rhythm and are influenced by downstream "pulling" forces generated by tissues in demand. The rest of this discussion focuses on laminar and turbulent flows as they have capacities to exert significant control over normal vascular dynamics and changes in them can drastically affect vascular pathologies. Continuous (unidirectional) laminar blood flow is uninterrupted and occurs at or near the capillary level and is characterized by layered flow in the absence of detectable flow velocity fluctuations or turbulence. Laminar flow is generally considered protective and beneficial for blood vessels and for maintenance of proper vascular tone, dilation, and tissue perfusion. Turbulent blood flow is associated with changes in the layered context of flow and is correlated with increased stresses on the vessel wall. Turbulent blood flow can be caused by branching or arborization of blood vessels (at bifurcations of arteries for example) and/or by intimal lesions or other luminal obstructions which create flow disturbances and turbulence. By its nature, turbulent blood flow is correlated with alterations in downstream perfusion and stress-induced changes in vessel architecture and mural wall remodeling. A schematic of laminar and turbulent blood flow is shown in Figure 3(a). Also shown are images from vascular Doppler ultrasound, a clinically-used non-interventional approach for estimating blood flow, vascular dimensions and lumen caliber, showing use of color flow systems to detect the na-

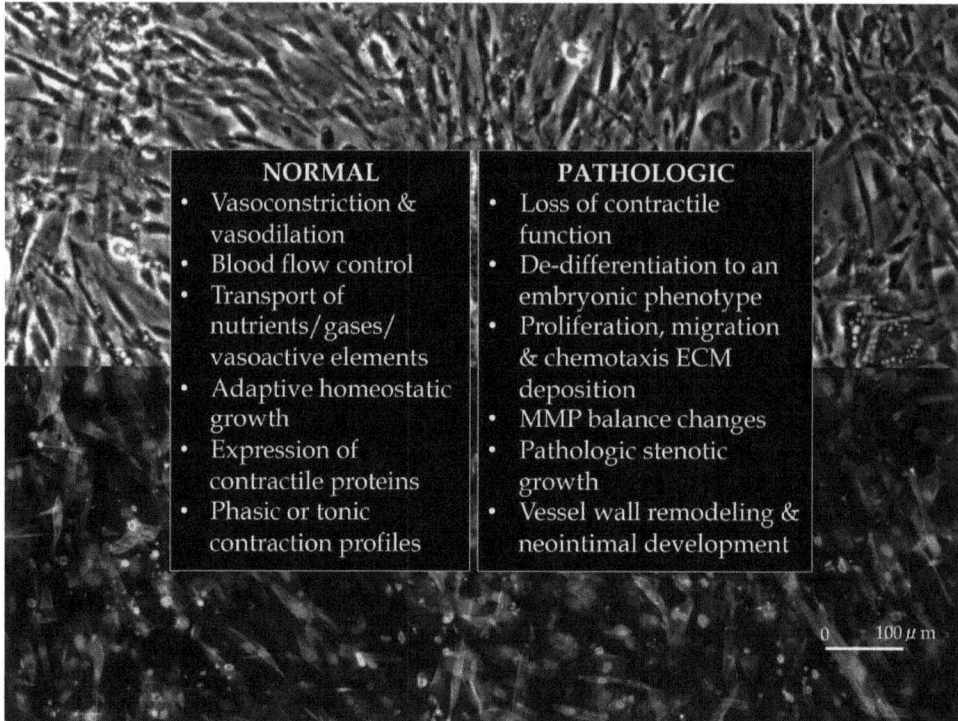

Figure 2: Normal or pathological arterial smooth muscle (ASM) phenotypes. Top image shows a photomicrograph of human coronary ASM cells at 100% confluence using inverted phase contrast microscopy and a 20x objective. Bottom image shows a fluorescent photomicrograph of the same human coronary ASM cells stained for G-actin and F-actin using specific probes conjugated to either Alexa Fluor (AF) 594 (red) or AF 488 (green), respectively. Cells were counterstained with DAPI (blue) in order to visualize nuclei. Scale bar shows 100 μm for both images. Insets list characteristics of normal versus pathologic phenotypes of ASM cells. Please refer to the online version for colored images for this figure.[3]

ture of arterial blood flow (b) and longitudinal arterial morphology showing arterial wall and luminal caliber (c).

Hemodynamics describes fluid-driven biophysical forces that govern many aspects of vascular function and that transport gases and metabolic fuels and nutrients. Driving pressure, transmural pressure, and hydrostatic pressure are important hemodynamic forces that regulate blood flow, and two major pressure-mediated forces are tensile wall stress and fluid shear stress. Tensile wall stress is the perpendicular force exerted by flowing blood on the vascular wall and represents forces due to distending blood pressure. Fluid shear stress is the force tangential to the vessel wall which corre-

---

[3] https://www.iconceptpress.com/book/coronary-artery-disease--causes-symptoms-and-treatments/11000164/1411001255/

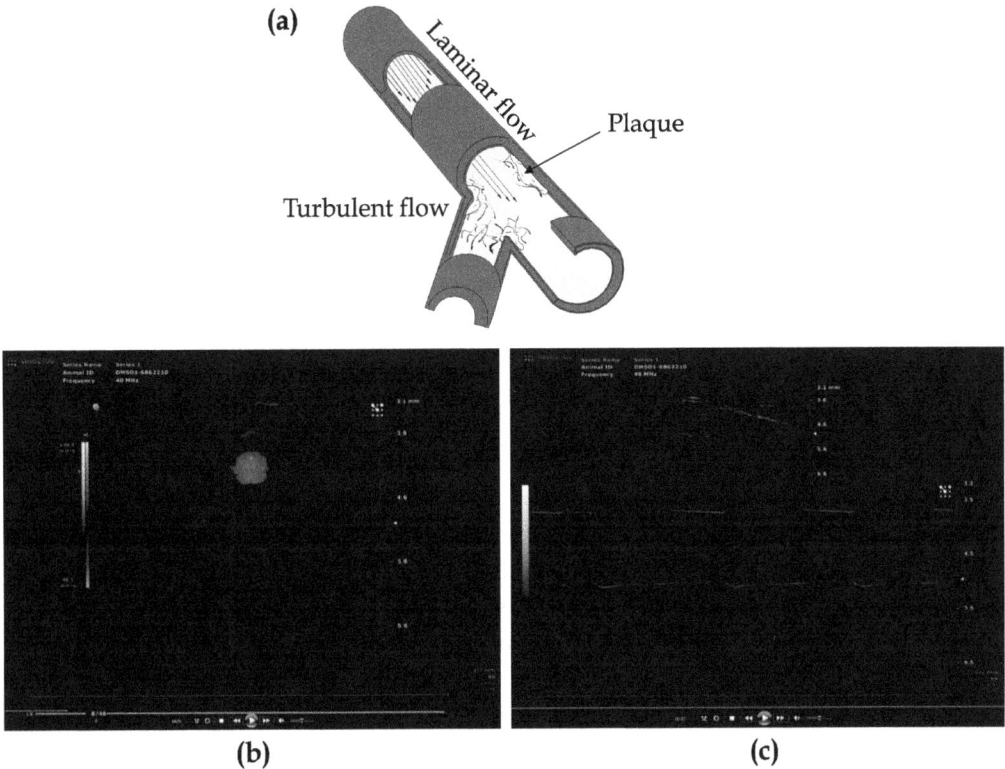

Figure 3: Hemodynamics: laminar versus turbulent blood flows. (a) Schematic of an artery cut-away showing normal upstream laminar blood flow depicted as parallel lines and turbulent blood flow resulting from a stenotic plaque at an arterial bifurcation depicted as multidirectional and mis-directed lines. (b) Using Doppler color flow systems (VisualSonics Vevo 2100) and carotid artery ultrasound, red color depicts blood flow towards the probe transducer (while blue color depicts blood flow away from the transducer). Through this approach one can detect laminar versus turbulent nature as well as magnitude of arterial blood flows. (c) Image represents longitudinal arterial ultrasound tracing showing carotid artery wall and lumen caliber. Episodic vessel expansion coincident with systolic arterial blood flow bolus is evident. Please refer to the online version for colored images for this figure.[4]

sponds to the frictional force of the blood in contact with the intimal surface (Davies *et al.*, 1992; White *et al.*, 2007). Changes in blood flow characteristics (i.e., from homeostatic laminar flow to disrupted turbulent flow) and/or alterations in flow-directed biophysical forces directly influence the vessel wall and can contribute markedly to the pathogenesis of CAD and CVD as described below.

---

[4] https://www.iconceptpress.com/book/coronary-artery-disease--causes-symptoms-and-treatments/11000164/1411001255/

4   Fundamentals of CAD

Coronary artery disease (CAD), otherwise known as coronary heart disease, is the most common form of heart disease and is a progressive pathology that affects the coronary circulation and that ultimately leads to partial or total vessel occlusion with compromised blood flow and hypoxia or anoxia in vital downstream tissues. This has clear clinical significance as it can lead to loss of oxygen and nutrient delivery to essential myocardium and accumulation of toxic byproducts of cellular metabolism, such as CO_2 and lactic acid. Atherosclerosis (from the Greek words *athero* (meaning gruel or paste) and *sclerosis* (hardness)) is a term used to describe the process of fatty substances, cholesterol, cellular waste products, calcium, fibrin, and other elements building up in the inner lining of an artery and has been determined to be a primary form of CAD. Atherosclerosis is characterized as a gradual, chronic, and cumulative disorder that involves inflammation, occlusive growth and remodeling of the vessel wall, and build-up of a stenotic atheroma or plaque. This multifactorial process is determined by congruent disorders of the immune, metabolic, circulatory, and vascular systems and includes dysfunction and/or fenestration of normal intimal endothelium and basement membrane, upregulation of vascular cell adhesion molecules, binding of low density lipoproteins to intimal proteoglycans, accumulation of lipids, cholesterol, calcium and cellular debris within the intima and sub-intimal space, macrophage and monocyte activation and formation of foam cells, activation and aggregation of localized platelets, and phenotypic modulation and uncontrolled proliferation of resident ASM cells (Crowther, 2005; Falk, 2006). Accordingly, the earliest visible lesion associated with atherosclerosis is a fatty streak of accumulated fat-laden foam cells in the intimal space. This process eventuates in a vicious and positive feedback cycle of inflammation and pathologic growth complete with luminal obstruction and development of a fibrous plaque, a hallmark of an established lesion. Unless otherwise jeopardized this plaque can remain stable for years, yet when it becomes unstable or compromised (via denudation of overlying endothelium and/or rupture) clinical symptoms often appear.

During the pathogenesis of atherosclerosis and other forms of stenotic CAD, ASM cells in the affected coronary circulation display a high degree of plasticity and switch from a normally quiescent and contractile phenotype to a growth-promoting, synthetic phenotype capable of robust proliferation, migration, and matrix production (Tulis, 2008; Gomez, 2012; Holt & Tulis, 2015; Tulis, 2015). During early stages of disease progression this phenotypic conversion occurs in response to locally secreted growth factors, mitogens and/or chemical attractants, circulating factors or hormones, or other vasoactive agents. Ensuing pathogenic processes can include stimulated cellular proliferation and DNA multiplication with polyploidy, aberrant cytokinesis with ensuing cellular hypertrophy, directed or ambiguous cellular migration and chemotaxis, altered matrix balance and MMP modulation via enhanced synthesis and secretion, and enhanced cellular necrosis and apoptosis. Concomitant events during this evolution phase can also include neovascularization of the growing plaque, calcium deposition and plaque mineralization, outward expansion of the affected vessel with compensatory luminal enlargement, and sustained inflammation. Combined, these elements of phenotypic switching of ASM cells and conversion or de-differentiation to an embryonic, growth-promoting phenotype are highly characteristic of disease pathology. Notably, considering its centrality in CAD pathogenesis and its potential to serve as a rate-limiting process for controlling disease maintenance and/or progression, abnormal ASM growth presents a critical target for attention in the study of CAD and CVD. Figure 4 shows photomicrographs of mechanically-injured and remodeled rat carotid arteries at high (a) and low (b) magnification. Figure 4(a) shows a hematoxylin and eosin-stained cross-section of an injured artery showing an enlarged adventitia, the medial wall and a newly formed and hyperplastic neointima. The external and internal elastic laminae are outlined in black. Figure 4(b) shows a Verhoeff/Van Giesen-stained injured artery cross-section with collagen-rich adventitia, an enlarged neointima, and a stenotic yet patent lumen.

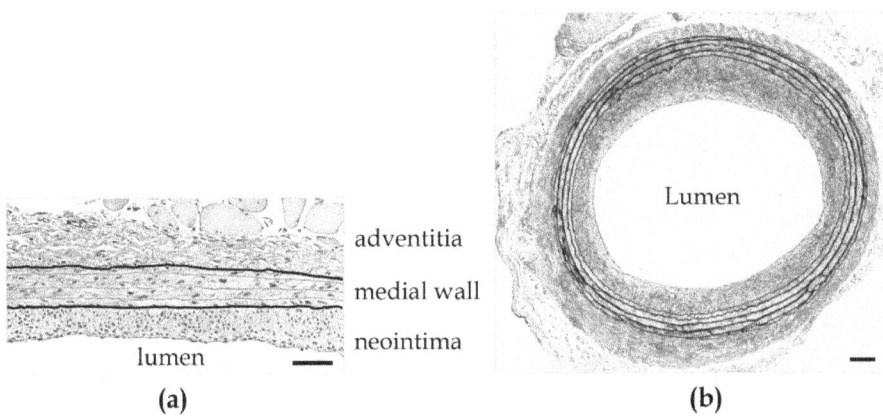

Figure 4: Pathologic arterial anatomy. **(a)** Photomicrograph of a hematoxylin and eosin-stained cross-section of a rat injured artery showing robust adventitia, medial wall, and the newly formed and hyperplastic neointima. The external and internal elastic laminae are outlined in black tracings. Scale bar in A is 80 μm. **(b)** Photomicrograph of Verhoeff/Van Giesen-stained rat injured artery cross-section with abundant advenititia, an enlarged neointima, and a stenotic but patent lumen. Scale bar in B is 50 μm. Please refer to the online version for colored images for this figure.[5]

5   Matrix Biology & ECM/MMP Balance

In addition to systemic inflammation, dysfunction of local AECs and de-differentiation and activation of local ASM cells, ECM remodeling is also a major contributor to phenotypic conversion underlying CAD pathogenesis. The predominant ECM constituents of

---

[5] https://www.iconceptpress.com/book/coronary-artery-disease--causes-symptoms-and-treatments/11000164/1411001255/

the arterial wall are collagen (mostly types I and III), elastin, fibronectin, and proteogly-cans, all of which are synthesized, secreted, and regulated by ASM. Endothelial cells are also major producers of basement membrane ECM proteins such as fibronectin, lam-inins, perlecan, and collagen types IV and XVIII (Jenkins *et al.*, 2007, Yin *et al.*, 2013). Da-vis and Senger (2005) published an elegant and detailed review on the roles of AECs and the ECM. Another known producer of ECM proteins are adventitial fibroblasts that interact with the resident medial ASM cells and modulate their phenotypic conversion and subsequent neointima formation and vascular remodeling (Saltore *et al.*, 2001). Fi-brillar collagen I, collagen IV, and laminin are all reported to promote the contractile phenotype of ASM under normal conditions (Thyberg & Hultgardh-Nilsson, 1994; Wang *et al.*, 2014). In CAD, however, activated ASM cells secrete elevated levels of all ECM-associated proteins, which then contribute to vessel wall remodeling, as well as matrix-degrading MMPs, whose activities can lead to reduced substrate adhesion and enhanced abilities of cells for proliferation and migration (Christensen *et al.*, 2010). The-se ECM proteins have also been reported to modulate ASM phenotype through binding to integrin receptors (Koyama *et al.*, 1998; Thyberg & Hultgardh-Nilsson, 1994). ASM cells are in direct contact with ECM proteins in the basement membrane, in internal and external elastic laminae, and in the interstitial matrix of vessel walls (Thyberg & Hultgardh-Nilsson, 1994). CAD involves remodeling of the vascular ECM through dy-namic inter-signaling processes between the vessel cells and the ECM, resulting in cellu-lar and ECM phenotypic changes which can lead to alterations in vessel wall diameter, stiffness, and function.

ASM cells synthesize collagens, particularly types I (the most abundant form in vessel walls) and III, which are excreted into the extracellular space where they self-assemble to form mature collagen fibrils. Predominantly, arterial collagen fibers align helically which allows them to structurally reinforce arteries in the circumferential and axial directions (Koyama *et al.*, 1996). As arterial pressures increase, helical collagen fi-bers change their alignment to become more circumferentially oriented, thereby adding to the circumferential mechanical properties of the artery (Amento *et al.*, 1991). During the disease process monomeric collagen I induces ASM cellular proliferation in re-sponse to growth factors including platelet derived growth factor (PDGF) and trans-forming growth factor (TGF)-β (Amento *et al.*, 1991; Davidson *et al.*, 1993), yet interest-ingly, polymerized collagen I is suggested to inhibit ASM proliferation due to upregula-tion of cyclin-dependent kinase 2 inhibitors (Koyama *et al.*, 1996).

In addition to collagen, several other ECM proteins are significant players in ASM matrix function and (patho)physiology. Fibronectin is an important modulator of vascu-lar wall structure and remodeling. In comparison to other ECM proteins that are more involved in the induction and maintenance of the contractile phenotype, under inimical conditions fibronectin stimulates ASM cell modulation towards a synthetic and prolif-erative phenotype elemental to CAD (Rohwedder *et al.*, 2012; Shi *et al.*, 2014). Fibron-ectin binds to collagen I through a well-characterized collagen-binding domain (Stef-fensen *et al.*, 1995). The peptide R1R2, which inhibits collagen I-fibronectin binding, when used in a vascular remodeling mouse model reduced neointimal development, inflammatory cell infiltration, and collagen I deposition in the vessel walls and maintained ASM cells in their contractile phenotype (Lee *et al.*, 2015). Hyaluronan, a gly-cosaminoglycan from the medial wall matrix, can enhance proliferation and migration of ASM cells (Evanko *et al.*, 1999) and its overexpression has been observed to accelerate the progression of atherosclerosis (Chai *et al.*, 2005). Hyaluronan synthesis, then, could be a viable target for reducing progression of CAD/CVD. The proteoglycans heparin and perlecan are major ECM regulators of ASM phenotype. Heparin reduces ASM cell proliferation and promotes the maintenance of a contractile phenotype (Hao *et al.*, 2002; Rensen *et al.*, 2007); however, the mechanisms by which heparin inhibits ASM proliferation are not fully understood. Perlecan inhibits ASM cell proliferation through its heparan sulphate side chains (Kinsella *et al.*, 2003), which have been suggested to sequester fibroblast growth factor-2 (Tran *et al.*, 2004). Of note, PDGF can down-regulate perlecan expression and thereby can reduce the influence of perlecan on ASM cell migration (Koyama *et al.*, 1998). Laminins are also an important component of the basement membrane and laminin-1, -5, -8, and -10 are all present in adult vasculature (Kingsley *et al.*, 2002; Welser, 2007). Laminin-5, for example, has been reported to enhance PDGF-B stimulated ASM cells proliferation and migration under stimulated, pathologic conditions (Kingsley *et al.*, 2002).

All these ECM-related factors are associated with modulation of ASM cells towards a synthetic phenotype underlying CAD, and many of these proteins have been suggested to be regulated by kinase signaling. Considering that Ser/Thr PKC-δ is involved in cellular proliferation and apoptosis (Fukumoto *et al.*, 1997; Leitges *et al.*, 2001), it was recently reported that PKC-δ deficiency results in reduced collagen I deposition in the media and adventitia of ASM cells (Lengfeld *et al.*, 2012). Fibrous atherosclerotic plaques are predominantly composed of collagen; therefore, tight regulation of collagen secretion and degradation is critical to vascular homeostasis as well as to the stability of an atherosclerotic plaque. Protein kinases, as regulators of vascular collagen, are promising drug targets for the treatment of CAD/CVD. Fibronectin can also be modulated by and serve as a modulator of protein kinases. While PKC-δ is necessary for induction of fibronectin synthesis by TGF-β (Ryer *et al.*, 2006), upregulation of fibronectin results in increased production of PKG linked to increased activity in contractile cells (Chamorro-Jorganes *et al.*, 2011). Also, the metabolic regulator AMPK has been shown to inhibit hyaluronan expression in human ASM cells (Vigetti *et al.*, 2011), yet in vivo studies are needed to examine the potential of AMPK as a hyaluronan-specific inhibitor of ASM activation. Additionally, we recently showed that AMPK has capacity to modulate TGF-β/Smad-mediated ASM proliferation and migration in the context of CAD (Stone *et al.*, 2015). Lastly, PKC-α expression has been shown to be blocked by a heparin-derived oligosaccharide in bovine ASM cells through G_0/G_1 cell cycle arrest and inhibited proliferation (Li *et al.*, 2012), and broad PKG inhibition decreased heparin effects in growth factor-activated ASM cells (Gilotti *et al.*, 2014).

Balancing matrix proteins are the family of MMP matrix-degrading enzymes. MMPs, secreted by inflammatory cells during CAD, influence the rates of atherogenesis and the stability of atherosclerotic plaques. The MMP family comprises 25 zinc-dependent proteinases that collectively can degrade every known ECM protein (Iyer *et al.*, 2014). MMP-1, MMP-3, MMP-8, and MMP-9 are highly expressed in atherosclerotic plaques and serum levels of MMP-1 and MMP-9 directly correlate with CAD severity (Newby, 2005; Tanindi *et al.*, 2011). Even though MMPs are mostly associated with rupture of arterial plaques by degradation of the plaque surface ECM, MMP-2, MMP-9, and MMP-14 stimulate migration and proliferation of ASM cells from the tunica media into the intima by degrading the ECM elements of the basement membrane (Dollery & Libby, 2006; Newby, 2006). This could potentially lead to increased plaque stability via enhanced cellular composition and thickening of the fibrous plaque. Huang and colleagues showed that PKC-βII activity induces neointimal expansion partially through increased MMP-9 expression (Huang *et al.*, 2010). Similarly, PKC-ε has been associated with MMP-2- and MMP-9-mediated ASM cell migration (Ding *et al.*, 2011). PKG suppresses MMP-2 expression and secretion in vitro (Dey & Lincoln, 2012), complementing some of our data showing that cyclic GMP/PKG signaling reduces expression and activity of both MMP-2 and MMP-9 in growth retardation of ASM in cultured cells and intact arteries (Tulis, 2008). Indeed, these findings strongly suggest mechanistic involvement of ECM proteins and ECM/MMP balance and their control by cyclic nucleotide-driven protein kinases in phenotypic modulation of ASM during CAD. Figure 5 (next page) shows a schematic depicting interaction between ECM proteins in an ASM cell and the resulting functional outcomes in CAD. Included are key intracellular and extracellular events and important signaling factors and processes that can serve critical roles in matrix balance. These include TGF-β and PDGF (and their respective receptors), important kinases such as PKC and PKG, structural matrix elements such as fibronectin, collagens, and laminin, and matrix-degrading MMPs. The figure also shows resulting functional outcomes in ASM phenotype (i.e., synthesis, proliferation, migration, contractility) foundational to structural changes and remodeling in the pathogenesis of CAD and CVD.

6   Cyclic Nucleotide-Driven Protein Kinase Signaling

Among the numerous molecular and cellular signaling pathways that serve to elicit control over cardiovascular functions, cyclic nucleotide signaling is of critical importance. Comprised primarily of the highly characterized canonical cyclic purine nucleotides cyclic AMP and cyclic GMP, this family of second messengers operates predominantly through downstream protein kinase signaling pathways to exert control over a wide variety of cellular processes. Cyclic AMP and cyclic GMP are firmly established as critical biological messengers in many mammalian tissues including ASM and this discussion focuses on their involvement during CAD.

It warrants mention that other cyclic purine nucleotides exist in the lesser known inosine 3′,5′-cyclic monophosphate (cyclic IMP) and xanthosine 3′,5′-cyclic monophosphate (cyclic XMP), and in fact these have been recently theorized as potentially serving second messenger roles (Beste & Seifert, 2013; Chen *et al.*, 2014); however, their involvement in ASM (patho)physiology and CAD and/or CVD has not yet been examined. An alternate family of cyclic pyrimidine nucleotides also exists and this includes cytidine 3′,5′-cyclic monophosphate (cyclic CMP), uridine 3′,5′-cyclic monophosphate (cy-

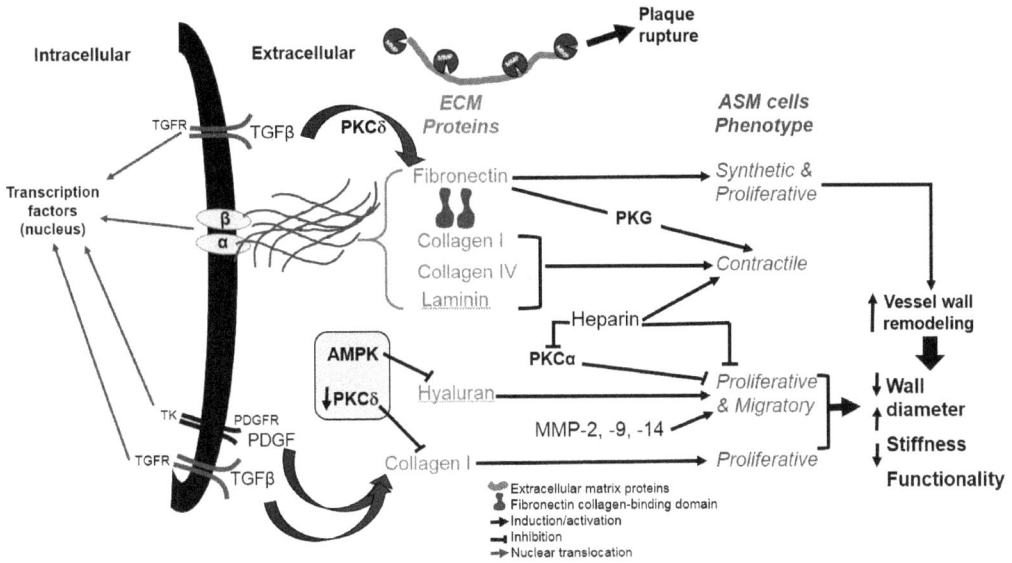

Figure 5: Effects of extracellular matrix (ECM) proteins and growth factors in the activation of arterial smooth muscle (ASM) cells and effects on vascular remodeling. Several ECM proteins (blue) can activate ASM cells through heterodimeric integrin receptors composed of α and β subunits (yellow) and modulate ASM phenotype either directly (block arrows) or by growth factor stimulation (curved arrows). Matrix metalloproteinases (MMPs) are commonly associated with atherosclerotic plaque rupture due to their roles in degrading vascular ECM, but some MMPs can also directly stimulate ASM proliferation and migration. AMPK and PKC-δ are specific inhibitors of ASM proliferative phenotype by respectively reducing hyaluran and collagen I levels. Red arrows denote nuclear translocation events that lead to changes in ASM cell phenotype foundational to CAD and CVD. Please refer to the online version for colored images for this figure.[6]

clic UMP), and thymidine 3′,5′-cyclic monophosphate (cyclic TMP) (Beste & Seifert, 2013; Bahre *et al.*, 2015); however, as with cyclic IMP and cyclic XMP their biological role(s) in ASM and CAD/CVD is unknown. Interestingly though and in relation to the AGC family of cyclic nucleotide-driven protein kinases (PK<u>A</u>, PK<u>G</u>, PK<u>C</u>), several of these 'alternate' cyclic nucleotides are thought to be synthesized through the same upstream machinery (Beste & Seifert, 2013; Chen *et al.*, 2014) and to utilize the same downstream kinases (Desch *et al.*, 2010) as cyclic AMP and cyclic GMP, pointing to the broad substrate specificity of cyclases and the diverse promiscuity and signaling cross-talk of downstream events.

Generation of cyclic AMP can occur through multiple avenues including adenylate cyclase (AC) stimulation by direct agonists or following β-stimulation or through G

---

[6] https://www.iconceptpress.com/book/coronary-artery-disease--causes-symptoms-and-treatments/11000164/1411001255/

protein-coupled receptor activation. Following AC stimulation, adenosine triphosphate (ATP) dephosphorylates to produce cyclic AMP and pyrophosphate (PPi). In similar fashion, following activation of guanylate cyclase (GC) through natriuretic peptides (which activate particulate GC) or by gaseous ligands (which activate soluble GC), guanosine triphosphate (GTP) is dephosphorylated to yield cyclic GMP and PPi. Detailed biomolecular mechanisms of cyclase-mediated cyclic AMP and cyclic GMP formation have been described (Tulis, 2008; Tulis, 2015). The preferred effector kinases, then, of cyclic AMP and cyclic GMP are the AGC kinases PKA and PKG, respectively (Arencibia et al., 2013). In addition to these canonical kinase pathways these cyclic nucleotides can also proceed through alternate kinase-directed pathways (Adderley et al., 2012a), direct ion channel modulation, or become degraded by specific members of the phosphodiesterase (PDE) family (Adderley et al., 2012b). In this light, conversion of cyclic AMP or GMP into inactive 5′-AMP or 5′-GMP is accomplished through specific PDEs that cleave the phosphodiester bonds of cAMP (by PDE-4, -7, -8) or cGMP (by PDE-5, -6, -9) to yield 5′-AMP or 5′-GMP. In turn, targeted PDE inhibition is capable of indirectly maintaining elevated levels of these cyclic nucleotides and their downstream kinases. In the mid to late 1980s this rationale was investigated as an approach to maintain kinase signaling for its potential treatment of CAD, but ironically this led to discovery of the PDE-5 inhibitor Sildenafil (Viagra), the most widely-prescribed oral agent for the treatment of erectile dysfunction (Briganti et al. 2005; Reffelmann et al. 2003). Our research team and others have provided evidence of promiscuity among many aspects of the cyclic AMP and cyclic GMP systems including 'cross-talk' between the activating cyclases, interactions between cyclic AMP/PKG, cyclic GMP/PKA and PKC, and non-selective PDE-directed kinase inactivation (discussed in detail below). Nonetheless, these intricate signaling cascades elicit a multitude of significant biological effects in ASM and are of critical importance in vascular physiology and pathology related to CAD and CVD. Figure 6 shows a schematic of cyclic GMP synthesis including up stream NO and CO cascades and downstream kinase-specific targets including cytoskeletal VASP fundamental to ASM (patho)physiology.

Protein kinases in general serve a wide variety of roles in a multitude of physiological and pathophysiological processes and represent one of the most ubiquitous, and functionally diverse families in the human genome constituting ~2% of all human genes with over 500 human protein kinases identified to date (Adderley et al., 2012a; Manning et al., 2002). Numerous kinase mutations have been identified in human diseases through genotype-phenotype analyses (Lahiry et al., 2010) and kinases have been theorized as instrumental therapeutic targets against CVD (Kompa & Krum, 2014; Wang et al., 2012). In fact, protein kinases already represent ~20% of all putative drug targets (Lahiry et al., 2010) and are likely the major pharmaceutical drug target of the 21st century (Cohen, 2002). More recently Dubey and colleagues (2015) showed 2-chloroadenosine (a stable adenosine analogue) increased cAMP levels and attenuated human coronary ASM cell proliferation which was reversed with PKA blockade. These recent findings highlight the relevance and timeliness of cyclic nucleotide dependent kinases currently being investigated as related to vascular growth disorders such as CAD.

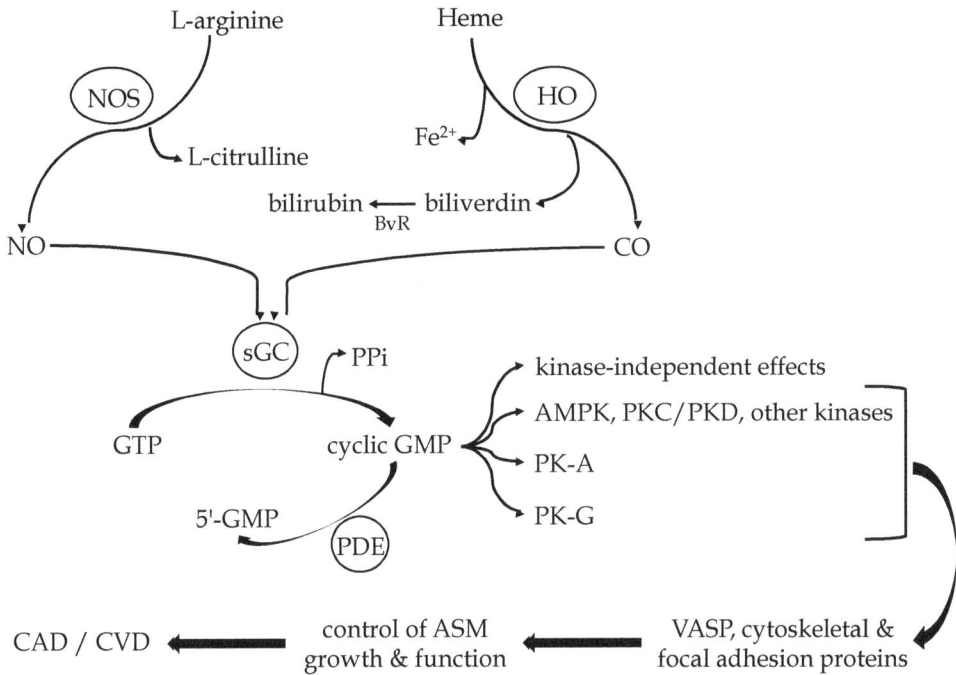

Figure 6: Signaling diagram for cyclic GMP synthesis and downstream signaling. Following upstream activation by a family of nitric oxide synthase (NOS) and/or heme oxygenase (HO) enzymes, L-arginine and heme, respectively, are metabolized to L-citrulline (with production of nitric oxide (NO)) and carbon monoxide (CO). These diatomic gases then activate soluble guanylate cyclase (sGC) which serves to dephosphorylate guanosine triphosphate (GTP) to yield cyclic GMP and pyrophosphate (PPi). Cyclic GMP is either degraded by a family of phosphodiesterases (PDE) or exerts downstream phosphorylative actions upon distinct kinases, primarily PKG, PKA and AMPK, as well as other kinases and non-kinase targets. The kinases can then act to regulate VASP and associated cytoskeletal/focal adhesion proteins which, in turn, helps to control aspects of arterial smooth muscle (ASM) growth and function as basic elements of CAD and/or CVD.

Several sub-families of kinases exist with a majority acting to phosphorylate either the -OH group of serine (Ser) and/or threonine (Thr) residues (the Ser/Thr kinases), which constitute about 80% of the total protein kinases (Manning *et al.*, 2002), or tyrosine (Tyr) residues (the Tyr kinases). For example, in regard to the Ser/Thr kinases, following binding of two cyclic AMP molecules to the regulatory subunit (dimer) of PKA a conformational change of this tetrameric enzyme occurs which causes release of its two catalytic subunits (Terrin *et al.* 2012). Active PKA goes on to phosphorylate proteins that have the motif Arginine-Arginine-X-Ser exposed, thereby phosphorylating and activating those targets. Like PKA, PKG as well as PKC/PKD and AMP kinase are all established Ser/Thr kinases that become activated through upstream substrate binding and phosphorylate a multitude of downstream targets. Additionally, some broad kinases act on all three amino acids (termed dual-specificity kinases), while lesser-known kinases can phosphorylate unique residues such as histidine (the His kinases) (Besant *et al.*, 2003).

PKA and PKG are select members among the more than 60 AGC kinases in the human genome and constitute the primary kinases acted upon by upstream cyclic AMP and cyclic GMP, respectively (Adderley, *et al.*, 2012a; Arencibia *et al.*, 2013; Pearce *et al.*, 2010). Through the act of site-specific (Ser/Thr or Tyr) and reversible phosphorylation of target proteins via phosphotransferase activity, these molecules exert potent signal transduction mechanisms which have capacity to control countless intracellular processes including many in ASM. Despite the ubiquitous nature and diversity of kinases in humans they share a common basic structure and mechanisms of action. Thorough comprehensive reviews have been published regarding cellular, biochemical and molecular mechanisms of protein kinases (Francis & Corbin, 1994; Adams, 2001; Ubersax & Ferrell, 2007; reviewed in Khalil, 2010), and herein only a succinct synopsis of key events is provided. Broadly speaking, protein kinases including members of the AGC family consist of a conserved catalytic domain of approximately 250 amino acids in length made up of one lobe of β-sheets in an N-terminus and a second lobe of α-helices in a C-terminus (Knighton *et al.*, 1991). Once ATP binds to a cleft between these two lobes (this constitutes the active site), a set of conserved residues within the catalytic domain transfers the terminal γ-phosphate of ATP to the hydroxyl oxygen of the receiving residue (Ser/Thr, Tyr) on the target (Francis & Corbin, 1994; Ubersax & Ferrell, 2007). This is followed by substrate release and removal of ADP from this active site and phosphorylation-driven activation or inactivation of the downstream target. Despite this common mechanism, kinase specificity is imparted by differences in hydrophobicity of surface residues, the overall charge of the enzyme, characteristics of the active site including the nature and sequence of ATP/substrate binding, rate-limiting steps, presence or absence of adapter or scaffolding proteins, and sub-cellular localization of the kinase.

Modification of target proteins via post-translational phosphorylation by any particular kinase can then dictate downstream enzyme and target protein expression and/or activities and downstream responses including those fundamental to aberrant cell proliferation and migration and matrix balance (i.e., phenotypic switching) that occurs in CAD pathogenesis. This is highly context-specific and can involve control of cell cycle progression by cyclins, cyclin-dependent kinases (CDKs), and/or CDK inhibitors, control of cell migration by cytoskeletal and focal adhesion elements including gap junctional connexins and VASP, and alterations in matrix balance including matrix proteins and/or degrading MMPs (Tulis, 2008; Mendelev *et al.*, 2009; Joshi *et al.*, 2011; Adderley *et al.*, 2012a; Adderley *et al.*, 2012b; Joshi *et al.*, 2012; Stone *et al.*, 2012; Stone *et al.*, 2013; Adderley *et al.*, 2015; Holt & Tulis, 2015; Joshi & Tulis, 2015; Stone *et al.*, 2015; Tulis, 2015). Additionally, kinase actions may be altered through modulation of dephosphorylating protein phosphatases (PPs) which have recently been theorized to serve regulatory roles in abnormal ASM growth (Stone *et al.*, 2012; Stone *et al.*, 2013).

Indeed, the downstream actions of kinase-driven phosphorylation events are wide-ranging and diverse and often paradoxical, resulting in target activation or inactivation in predominantly context-specific manner (Adderley *et al.*, 2012a; Ubersax & Ferrell, 2007).

Given the centrality of cyclic nucleotide and cyclic nucleotide-driven protein kinase signaling in ASM physiology and pathology, brief discussion is warranted for their roles in mediating the critical functions of vascular contraction and relaxation. As discussed above, during the pathogenesis of CAD and CVD, ASM undergoes a loss of its contractile capabilities and undergoes a phenotypic reversal to an embryonic, growth-promoting, and synthetic form. Thus, a common thread of cyclic nucleotide/kinase action in ASM phenotypic modulation is the ability of these agents to elegantly regulate smooth muscle tone. Although detailed mechanisms have been previously described (reviewed in Gao *et al.*, 2001; Webb, 2003; Khalil, 2010), generally speaking in ASM under normal conditions, following agonist stimulation intracellular calcium ($[Ca^{2+}_i]$) rises and binds calmodulin (CaM), which in turn activates the Ser/Thr myosin light chain kinase (MLCK). Activated MLCK then phosphorylates Ser19 of the 20 kD regulatory myosin light chain (MLC), which activates myosin ATPase activity and initiates actin-myosin crossbridge formation and subsequent crossbridge cycling central to ASM contraction (Gao *et al.*, 2001). Calcium-independent smooth muscle contraction can also occur following agonist stimulation of inositol triphosphate (IP3), which in turn activates RhoA (RhoA-GTP) which then binds to and activates ROCK, leading to phosphorylation and inhibition of MLC phosphatase and reduced capacity to dephosphorylate MLC (Surks, 2007). In general, inactivation of crossbridge cycling and cessation of smooth muscle contraction occurs via dephosphorylation of the MLC through actions of MLC phosphatase.

Regarding cyclic nucleotide-directed kinase control of ASM contraction, PKG stimulation promotes vascular relaxation through several mechanisms (Surks, 2007). PKG directly inhibits the mobilization of $[Ca^{2+}_i]$, thereby preventing calcium-CaM-mediated activation of MLCK (Cornwell & Lincoln, 1989). PKG can open calcium-activated potassium channels, thereby leading to cell hyperpolarization and relaxation (Archer *et al.*, 1994). PKG can also operate via a calcium-independent mechanism by activating MLC phosphatase and dephosphorylating MLC (Lee *et al.*, 1997). Cyclic AMP-driven PKA shares these avenues for controlling ASM contraction through reduction in $[Ca^{2+}_i]$, direct and indirect (via enhanced MLC phosphatase) modes for inhibiting MLC phosphorylation, and stimulation of calcium-activated potassium channels and resulting hyperpolarization. Moreover, both PKA and PKG have been found to promote vasorelaxation via phosphorylation of Ser16 on the small heat shock-related protein (Hsp) 20, which appears to alter actin-myosin relations, crossbridge formation, and actin-focal adhesion dynamics necessary for contraction (Somara *et al.*, 2010; Woodrum *et al.*, 2003). Lastly, considering kinase promiscuity among AGC kinase family members (Adderley *et al.*, 2012a), brief discussion is warranted for PKC in vascular contraction. In smooth muscle PKC exists in the calcium-dependent forms α and β and in the calcium-independent forms ε and ζ, and both of these groups of isoforms have been implicated in PKC-mediated vascular contraction (Andrea & Walsh, 1992; Khalil, 2010). PKC can operate to induce contraction by increasing myofilament force sensitivity to [Ca^{2+}]$_i$, through calcium/CaM-mediated activation of MLCK and induction of MLC phosphorylation, and by establishing actin-myosin interactions (Rasmussen *et al.*, 1987; Khalil, 2010). PKC has also been observed to induce smooth muscle contraction in calcium-independent fashion by phosphorylating the actin-associated filament calponin, thereby reducing its affinity for F-actin and alleviating its inhibition of crossbridge cycling (Horowitz *et al.*, 1996; Walsh *et al.*, 1996).

Serving as an 'off switch' to balance kinase-driven phosphorylation is a family of enzymatic PPs. Removal of a phosphate group from kinase-targeted proteins by PPs serves to moderate cell signaling and helps to regulate many cellular processes involved in differentiation, proliferation, migration, apoptosis, and embryonic development. Similar to amino acid specificity of the kinases, there exist specific Ser/Thr PPs and specific Tyr PPs that balance the actions of Ser/Thr and Tyr kinases, respectively. Following activation of the kinases via upstream signals, they target downstream substrate proteins in a cell- and tissue-specific fashion. We recently documented ability of both global PPs and Ser/Thr PPs in conjunction with activated upstream PKA, PKG and/or AMP kinase signals to elicit control over deleterious ASM proliferation and migration (Stone *et al.*, 2012; Stone *et al.*, 2013).

Recent discoveries using pharmacology, over-expressing and deficient transgenic models, and site-specific modulation of targeted residues have revealed signaling promiscuity and lack of precision for both upstream modes of kinase activation and for downstream phosphorylated targets (Worner *et al.*, 2007; Tulis, 2008; Mendelev *et al.*, 2009; Desch *et al.*, 2010; Joshi *et al.*, 2011; Adderley *et al.*, 2012a; Stone *et al.*, 2012; Beste & Seifert, 2013; Chen *et al.*, 2014; Tulis, 2015). While Ser/Thr and Tyr kinases generally act on their preferred substrates, these enzymes are also attracted to residues that flank both sides of the phosphoacceptor site (the Ser, Thr and/or Tyr); thus, the catalytic cleft of the kinase interacts not only with its preferred Ser, Thr or Tyr phosphoacceptor but also with their flanking regions, thereby binding to common recognition sequences among similar substrate family members and in turn reducing kinase specificity. This kinase crosstalk or promiscuity affords broad impact of upstream kinase signals but at the same time lends difficulty in ascertaining precise downstream signaling mechanisms and targets. Among the numerous bioactive targets of the AGC kinases PKA, PKG, and PKC that also serve as a target for their promiscuous signaling is the focal adhesion protein VASP.

7   VASP

Cellular migration or chemotaxis in response to pathologic cues or tissue damage relies heavily on reorganization of the actin cytoskeleton that is mediated by an array of focal adhesion adapter proteins. One of these proteins that is essential for this reorganization to occur and that predominantly acts as a substrate for many cyclic nucleotide-driven kinases is vasodilator-stimulated serum phosphoprotein or VASP. VASP, a member of the Ena/VASP Homology (EVH) family of closely-related proteins, serves critical functions in cytoskeletal stability and dynamics that are involved in intracellular signaling pathways regulating integrin-ECM interactions. VASP is comprised of an N-terminal EVH1 domain (used to target focal adhesion and membrane domains), a mid-region that binds to Src-homology 3 (SH3) domains and tryptophan-rich WW domain-containing proteins that aid in Ser/Thr binding, and a C-terminal EVH2 domain that mediates tetramerization (a right-handed coiled coil with 15 residue repeats) and actin/focal adhesion binding. Originally characterized as a substrate for cyclic nucleotide-directed phosphorylation signals (Reinhard *et al.*, 2001; Krause *et al.*, 2002) with PKA acting preferentially on VASP$_{Ser157}$ and PKG acting primarily on VASP$_{Ser239}$ (Chen *et al.*, 2004; Worner *et al.* 2007), to date at least four distinct Ser/Thr phosphorylation sites have been identified on VASP: Ser$_{157}$, Ser$_{239}$, Thr$_{278}$, Ser$_{322}$ (Butt *et al.*, 1994; Chitaley *et al.*, 2004; Thomson *et al.*, 2011). Interestingly, more recent studies have observed crosstalk and lack of specificity of these and other Ser/Thr kinases to phosphorylate discrete residues on VASP. Notably, recent findings from our laboratory in commercial (Mendelev *et al.*, 2009) and primary (Joshi *et al.*, 2011; Adderley *et al.*, 2012a; Adderley *et al.*, 2012b; Adderley *et al.*, 2015; Tulis, 2008; Tulis, 2015) ASM cells documents ability of cyclic AMP and cyclic GMP to not only communicate with their respective canonical PKA and PKG targets but to also target other kinases as well. We have observed that cyclic AMP, stimulated both directly and indirectly, induces PKG in addition to PKA and phosphorylates both the reported PKG target VASP$_{Ser239}$ and the accepted PKA target VASP$_{Ser157}$. Likewise, we have stimulated cyclic GMP, directly and indirectly, and have found stimulation of PKG and PKA as well as both VASP$_{Ser239}$ and VASP$_{Ser157}$. We have also observed both cyclic AMP and cyclic GMP have capacity to stimulate members of the diverse PKC/PKD family (Adderley *et al.*, 2012a). Considering other kinases, we recently reported that the Ser/Thr metabolic gauge AMP kinase, traditionally thought to act uniquely on its regulatory site VASP$_{Thr278}$ (Blume *et al.*, 2007), also has capacity to phosphorylate VASP$_{Ser157}$ yet does not significantly affect VASP$_{Ser239}$ (Stone *et al.*, 2012; Stone *et al.*, 2013). Lastly, it was reported that PKC-driven PKD, another Ser/Thr kinase involved in extracellular receptor-mediated signal transduction, phosphorylates both its reported VASP$_{Ser322}$ as well as VASP$_{Ser157}$ (Doppler *et al.*, 2013). A schematic of the primary structure of VASP with essential EVH1 and EVH2 domains, the SH3- and WW-domain binding region, and preferred (but not exclusive) sites of action for select Ser/Thr protein kinases (adapted from Madej *et al.*, 2014) is shown in Figure 7.

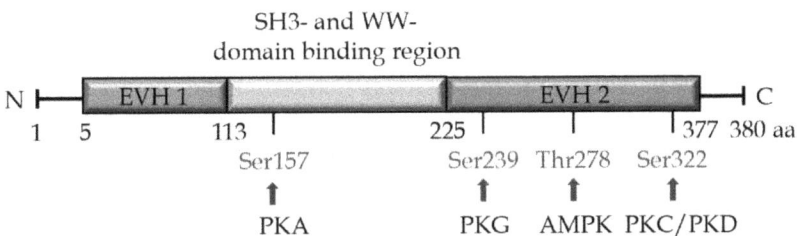

Figure 7: Linear primary structure for VASP with EVH1 and EVH2 domains and preferred Ser/Thr sites for select kinase action.

Functionally, VASP operates as an anti-capping protein and promoter of actin polymerization by delivering monomeric globular (G) actin to the barbed end of growing filamentous (F) actin (Barzik *et al.*, 2005; Bear *et al.*, 2002; Breitsprecher *et al.*, 2008). Therefore, when VASP is inhibited (or phosphorylated), it can no longer drive F-actin formation and actin-mediated cell motility. Instead, phosphorylated (inactivated) VASP promotes cytostasis by keeping the G-actin pool elevated (Stone *et al.*, 2012). If total actin protein expression (β-actin) remains unchanged, then quantifying the G:F actin ratio as an estimate of the balance of depolymerized:polymerized actin serves to describe the migratory status of adherent cells since the cellular actin is either depolymerizing or polymerizing in the context of cellular movement or migration. Actin polymerization and leading edge formation are essential for directional cellular movement and migration or chemotaxis, and VASP operates in support of these cytoskeletal rearrangements necessary for cell movement. Site-specific phosphorylation of VASP (at one or more of its aforementioned Ser/Thr residues) acts to inhibit its anti-capping potential and in turn serves to reduce actin polymerization and inhibit or prevent migration (Blume *et al.*, 2007). VASP also acts as a regulator of platelet function and adhesion as well as in cytoskeletal dynamics and processes such as cell adhesion and proliferation (Adderley *et al.*, 2012a; Adderley *et al.*, 2015; Cheng *et al.*, 2014; Henes *et al.*, 2009; Kwiatkowski *et al.*, 2003). VASP is also suggested to have anti-tumorigenic properties (Doppler *et al.*, 2013) and anti-inflammatory actions in diabetes (Cheng *et al.*, 2014). In the context of CAD and CVD, we have recently examined VASP and its phosphorylated forms and their abilities to control migration of commercial, rat primary, and human coronary ASM cells. Cumulative findings show that the reported PKA target VASP$_{Ser157}$ and the AMPK target VASP$_{Thr278}$ generally act to reduce cellular proliferation while the PKG site VASP$_{Ser239}$ as well as VASP$_{Thr278}$ work to inhibit migration (Adderley *et al.*, 2012a; Mendelev *et al.*, 2008; Joshi *et al.*, 2013; Stone *et al.*, 2012; Stone *et al.*, 2013). In complement, other investigators reported recently that the PKC/PKD residue VASP$_{Ser322}$ also controls cellular migration (Doppler *et al.*, 2013). In whole, results show strong support for differential VASP species in serving crucial functions to control pathologic proliferation and migration in the context of CAD. Certainly, VASP as a target of cyclic nucleotide-directed kinase signals holds great promise regarding its ability to control deleterious ASM growth that underlies significant pathologies such as CAD and CVD.

8   Pharmacologic Cyclic GMP Agonists

Despite clear significance and utility, there have been numerous concerns raised for both nitric oxide (NO)- and carbon monoxide (CO)-mediated cyclic GMP signals including reaction with molecular oxygen, thiols and transition metal ions, development of reactive species, modification of lipids, proteins and nucleic acids, and reduced efficacy via tolerance and/or tachyphylaxis following prolonged clinical treatment, and limited or restricted bioactivity (Davis *et al.*, 2001; Andrews *et al.*, 2002; Gori & Parker, 2002). These drawbacks, in turn, have warranted discovery of alternate routes for activating Ser/Thr kinases and their associated targets including VASP (all downstream of

NO/CO) in efforts to identify novel and potentially beneficial therapies devoid of such drawbacks. In this light, two families of synthetic sGC/cyclic GMP agonists have been developed that lack known limitations of traditional NO/CO signaling and that have capacity to serve as alternate routes for activating cyclic nucleotide signals in ASM (reviewed in Jackson *et al.*, 2007; Tulis, 2008; Tulis, 2015). Heme-dependent sGC stimulators depend on a functional (reduced) cyclase heme in order to enhance enzyme activity and cyclic GMP synthesis. Thus, under settings where the cyclase heme is removed or rendered dysfunctional these agents lose their activity and become inactive or less active. Heme-independent sGC activators, by comparison, maintain functionality under heme-deficient or -oxidized conditions and therefore are considered more therapeutically advantageous for diseased or injured tissues as occurs in CAD/CVD. Table 1 shows examples of some known stimulators and activators of sGC/cyclic GMP.

sGC / cyclic GMP stimulators	sGC / cyclic GMP activators
A-350619	BAY 58-2667
BAY 41-2272	BAY 60-2770
BAY 41-8543	HMR-1766
BAY 51-9491	S-3448
BAY 60-4552	
BAY 63-2521	
YC-1	

Table 1: Examples of some known stimulators and activators of sGC and cyclic GMP.

Much work from our lab over the past few years has focused on the abilities of these stimulators and activators to elicit control over ASM growth in the context of CAD/CVD using a variety of experimental platforms. YC-1 [3-(5'-hydroxymethyl-2'-furyl)-1-benzyl indazole], one of the originally characterized sGC stimulators (Ko *et al.*, 1994; Wu *et al.*, 1995), has been documented to elicit anti-platelet, anti-proliferative, anti-synthetic and pro-apoptotic growth-mitigating properties in ASM using in vitro, ex vivo and in vivo experimental models (Tulis *et al.*, 2000; Tulis *et al.*, 2002; Tulis, 2004; Keswani *et al.*, 2009; Liu *et al.*, 2009). More recently a next generation sGC stimulator and YC-1 mimetic BAY 41-2272 [(5-cyclo-propyl-2-[1-(2-fluorobenzyl)-1*H*-pyrazolo[3,4-*b*]pyridine-3-yl]-pyrimidin-4-ylamine)] (Becker *et al.*, 2001; Stasch *et al.*, 2001) was shown to induce PKG and PKA signaling and downstream VASP phosphorylation and to control ASM growth including regulation of matrix/MMP balance (Mendelev *et al.*, 2009; Joshi *et al.*, 2011; Adderley *et al.*, 2012a; Adderley *et al.*, 2012b). Interestingly, adding to the aforementioned promiscuity of cyclic nucleotide-driven kinase signaling, pharmacologic blockade studies reveal that BAY 41-2272 possess divergent downstream actions on cellular proliferation versus cellular migration (Joshi *et al.*, 2011; Adderley *et al.*, 2012a).

Lastly, using the heme-independent sGC activator BAY 60-2770 [4-({(4-carboxybutyl)[2-(5-fluoro-2-{[4'-(trifluoromethyl)biphenyl-4-yl]methoxy}phenyl)ethyl]   amino}methyl) benzoic acid] (BAY60; a kind gift from Bayer HealthCare, Germany) in rat primary ASM cells, rat commercial (A7r5) ASM cells, and human coronary ASM cells we have observed it to act primarily on cyclic GMP and PKG (with minimal influence on cyclic AMP/PKA), to phosphorylate both $VASP_{Ser239}$ and $VASP_{Ser157}$, to elicit control of ASM via cytoskeletal rearrangement quantified by G:F actin, and to reduce cellular proliferation and migration as well as injury-induced neointimal formation and vessel wall remodeling. Figure 8 (next page) shows some of these observations in human coronary ASM cells: (a) demonstrates that BAY60 (0.1-10 µM) significantly increases PKG activity compared to vehicle controls after 60 minutes using an ELISA-based activity assay (Cyclex); (b) shows that BAY60 dose-dependently reduces cell proliferation after 24 hours compared to vehicle (Veh) controls; (c, d) show preliminary results suggesting that BAY60 (10 µM) increases G:F actin ratio compared to Veh controls after 60 minutes, indicative of a more stable cytoskeletal phenotype and reduced capacity for proliferation and migration (Stone *et al.*, 2013). Indeed, these early findings using the heme-independent sGC activator BAY60 in human coronary ASM cells (and rat primary tissues) support a role for cyclic nucleotide-directed kinases in controlling aberrant ASM growth as an underpinning of CAD.

9   Summary & Future Directions

Coronary artery disease and CVD remain the number one cause of morbidity and mortality in the United States and worldwide and is associated with staggering economic costs as well. Notwithstanding major advances in our knowledge of the underlying mechanisms of these disorders and significant progress in our strategies aimed at their control, all estimates suggest an increasing trend in their prevalence over the next several decades. In our never-ending struggle to understand key elements behind normal vascular biology as well as regulatory mechanisms that underlie vascular pathology, we must continue to make pivotal inroads into potential routes for controlling and/or eliminating these dreaded disorders. It is generally thought that many, if not all, of the causes behind CAD/CVD are preventable and that future endeavors should focus on prevention strategies and early diagnoses and intervention to combat these diseases (AHA), 2011). In cumulative efforts to identify and characterize key elements behind CAD and CVD, we and others have focused our basic and clinical efforts at gaining more thorough understanding of the vital roles for ASM and the multifunctional cyclic nucleotide and cyclic nucleotide-directed kinase signals discussed herein. In our mind these represent highly promising yet incompletely understood targets capable of controlling pathologic vascular growth that accompanies vascular disease. Only through determined basic and clinical investigation can we hope to better understand crucial aspects of vascular biology and pathology and in that, gain insights into our seemingly unrelenting struggle against CAD and CVD.

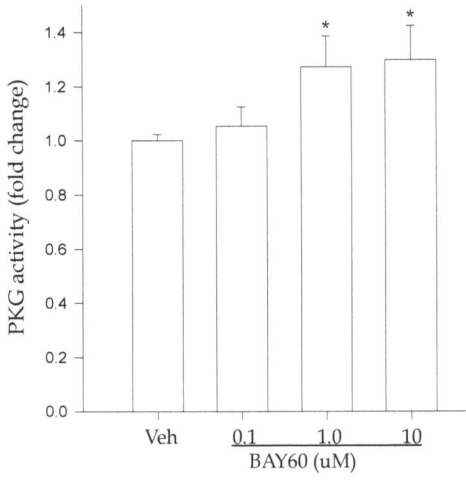

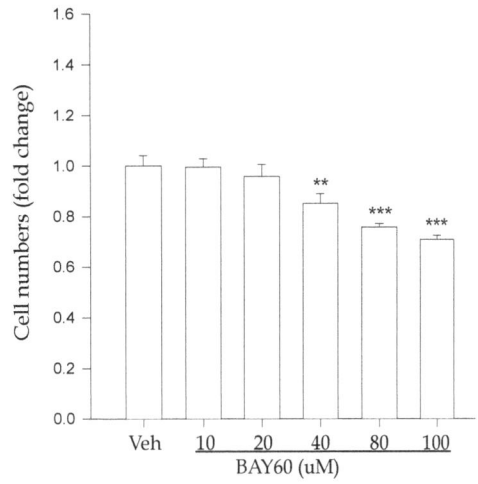

(a)

(b)

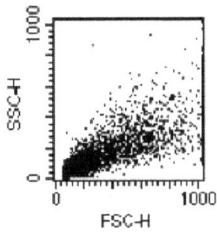

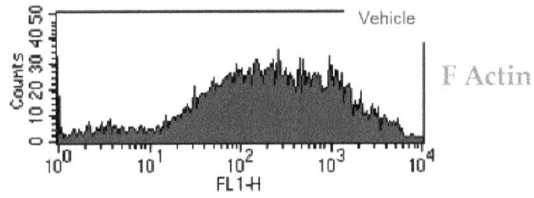

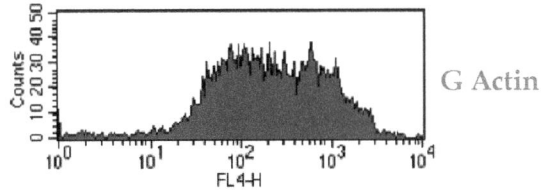

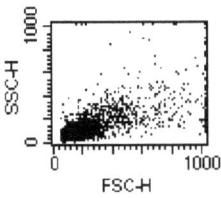

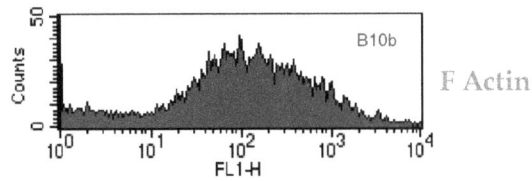

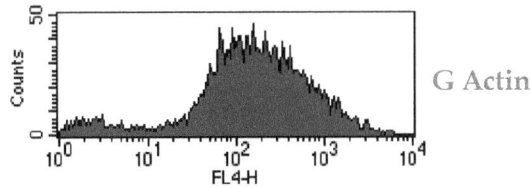

(c)

Continued on next page…

... Continued from previous page

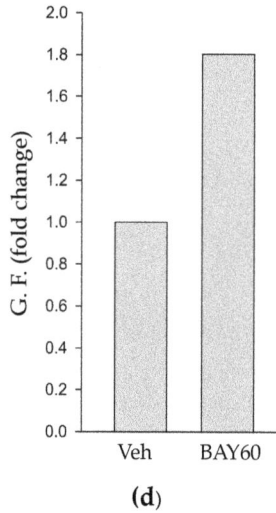

(d)

Figure 8: Kinase activity and growth retardation by the heme-independent sGC activator BAY 60-2770 (BAY60) in human coronary ASM cells. Cells were treated with vehicle (Veh) or BAY60 and assayed for PKG activity and cell proliferation. **(a)** After 60 min BAY60 elicited a significant, dose-dependent (~ 30%) increase in PKG activity compared to Veh. No observable changes were found in PKA activity following BAY60 treatment (data not shown). **(b)** After 24 hours cell numbers were estimated using DNA quantification, and BAY60 elicited a significant, dose-dependent reduction in cell numbers (through 100 μM) compared to Veh controls. $*p < 0.05$, $**p < 0.01$, $***p < 0.001$ versus Veh. Preliminary results also suggest that BAY60 increases G-actin to F-actin ratio in human coronary ASM cells. Cells were treated with Veh or BAY60 (10 μM) for 60 min, after which cells were trypsinized and stained for G or F actin using deoxyribonuclease I and phalloidin, respectively, conjugated to Alexa Fluor 594 (red for G-actin) or 488 (green for F-actin). Using the same morphology (forward/side scatter) gate for each run, at least 10,000 cells per group were analyzed using the BD FACSVantage high-speed cell sorter. Quantification of G:F ratio was performed by dividing the mean G-actin by the mean F-actin fluorescent intensities. **(c)** shows representative scatter plots for F-actin and G-actin for both the Veh (upper panels) and the BAY60 (lower panels) groups, while quantification in **(d)** reveals an 80% increase in G:F following BAY60 treatment compared to Veh controls. Please refer to the online version for colored images for this figure.[7]

---

[7] https://www.iconceptpress.com/book/coronary-artery-disease--causes-symptoms-and-treatments/11000164/1411001255/

Acknowledgements

We would like to acknowledge our many colleagues who are also engaged in this exciting yet often perplexing area of study as well as the many investigators who have significantly contributed to the fields of cyclic nucleotide and kinase signaling and the cardiovascular sciences but whose works were not cited in this chapter due to formatting limits. This work was supported by the Chapter 33 Post 9/11 GI Bill, award number R01HL81720 from the National Heart, Lung, and Blood Institute (NHLBI), National Institutes of Health (NIH), award number 14SDG1886005 from the AHA, an ECU Brody School of Medicine Seed/Bridge Grant, and a Brody Brothers Endowment Fund Award. This content is solely the responsibility of the authors and does not necessarily represent the official views of the AHA, NHLBI, NIH, ECU and/or the Brody Brothers Endowment Fund.

List of abbreviations

AC   adenylate cyclase

AECs   arterial endothelial cells

AGC kinases   protein kinase A, protein kinase G, protein kinase C

AHA   American Heart Association

AMPK AMP-activated protein kinase

ASM   arterial smooth muscle

ATP   adenosine triphosphate

BAY 41-2272   (5-cyclopropyl-2-[1-(2-fluorobenzyl)-1*H*-pyrazolo[3,4-*b*]pyridine- 3-yl]-pyrimidin-4-ylamine

BAY 60-2770   4-({(4-carboxybutyl)[2-(5-fluoro-2-{[4'-(trifluoromethyl)biphenyl- 4-yl]methoxy}phenyl) ethyl]amino}methyl)benzoic acid

$[Ca^{2+}_i]$ intracellular calcium

CAD   coronary artery disease

CaM   calmodulin

CO   carbon monoxide

CO2   carbon dioxide

CVD   cardiovascular disease

cyclic AMP   3′,5′-cyclic adenosine monophosphate

cyclic CMP   cytidine 3′,5′-cyclic monophosphate

cyclic GMP   3′,5′-cyclic guanosine monophosphate

cyclic IMP   inosine 3′,5′-cyclic monophosphate

cyclic TMP   thymidine 3′,5′-cyclic monophosphate

cyclic UMP   uridine 3′,5′-cyclic monophosphate

cyclic XMP   xanthosine 3′,5′-cyclic monophosphate

DNA   deoxyribonucleic acid

ECM   extracellular matrix

EVH   Ena/VASP homology

F-actin filamentous actin

GC   guanylate cyclase
G:F   G-actin:F-actin ratio
His   histidine
Hsp   heat shock-related protein
IP3   inositol triphosphate
MLC   myosin light chain
MLCK   myosin light chain kinase
MMP   matrix metalloproteinase
NHLBI   National Heart, Lung, and Blood Institute
NIH   National Institutes of Health
NO   nitric oxide
PDE   phosphodiesterase
PDGF   platelet derived growth factor
PDGFR   platelet derived growth factor receptor
pGC   particulate guanylate cyclase
PKA   cyclic AMP-dependent protein kinase (or protein kinase A)
PKC   protein kinase C
PKD   protein kinase D
PKG   cyclic GMP-dependent protein kinase (or protein kinase G)
PPi   pyrophosphate
PPs   protein phosphatases
Ser   serine
sGC   soluble guanylate cyclase
SH3   Src-homology 3
TGF   transforming growth factor
TGFR   transforming growth factor receptor
TK   tyrosine kinase
Thr   threonine
Tyr   tyrosine
VASP   vasodilator-stimulated serum phosphoprotein
Veh   vehicle (control)
YC-1   3-(5'-hydroxymethyl-2'-furyl)-1-benzyl indazole

References

Adams, J.A. (2001). Kinetic and catalytic mechanisms of protein kinases. Chem. Rev. 101: 2271–2290.

Adderley, S.P., Joshi, C.N., Martin, D.N., Mooney, S., Tulis, D.A. (2012a). Multiple Kinase Involvement in the Regulation of Vascular Growth, Advances in Protein Kinases, Ch. 6, pp. 131–150, Ed. G. Da Silva Xavier, InTech Open Access Publishers, ISBN 978-953-51-0633-3.

Adderley, S.P., Joshi, C.N., Martin, D.N., Tulis, D.A. (2012b). *Phosphodiesterases regulate BAY 41-2272-induced VASP phosphorylation in vascular smooth muscle cells. Front. Pharmacol. 3:10.doi: 10.3389/fphar.201200010.*

Adderley, S.P., Martin, D.N., Tulis, D.A. (2015). *Exchange protein activated by cAMP (EPAC) controls migration of vascular smooth muscle cells in concentration- and time-dependent manner. Arch. Physiol. 2:2.doi: 10.7243/2055-0898-2-2; http://www.hoajonline.com/journals/pdf/2055-0898-2-2.pdf.*

Amento, E.P., Ehsani, N., Palmer, H., Libby, P. (1991). *Cytokines and growth factors positively and negatively regulate interstitial collagen gene expression in human vascular smooth muscle cells. Arterioscler. Thromb. Vasc. Biol. 11: 1223–1230.*

American Heart Association, on behalf of the American Heart Association Advocacy Coordinating Committee, Stroke Council, Council on Cardiovascular Radiology and Intervention, Council on Clinical Cardiology, Council on Epidemiology and Prevention, Council on Arteriosclerosis, Thrombosis and Vascular Biology, Council on Cardiopulmonary, Critical Care, Perioperative and Resuscitation, Council on Cardiovascular Nursing, Council on the Kidney in Cardiovascular Disease, Council on Cardiovascular Surgery and Anesthesia, and Interdisciplinary Council on Quality of Care and Outcomes Research. (2011). *Forecasting the future of cardiovascular disease in the United States. Circulation 123:933–944. doi: 10.1161/CIR.0b013e31820a55f5.*

American Heart Association, on behalf of the American Heart Association Statistics Committee and Stroke Statistics Subcommittee. (2014). *Heart Disease and Stroke Statistics – 2014 Update. Circulation 129: e28–e292; doi: 10.1161/01.cir. 0000441139.02102.80.*

Andrea, J.E., Walsh, M.P. (1994). *Protein kinase C of smooth muscle. Hypertension 20: 585–595.*

Andrews, K.L., Triggle, C.R., Ellis, A. (2002). *NO and the vasculature: where does it come from and what does it do? Heart Fail. Rev. 7: 423–45.*

Archer, S.L., Huang, J.M.C., Hampl, V., Nelson, D.P., Shultz, P.J., Weir, E.K. (1994). *Nitric oxide and cGMP cause vasorelaxation by activation of a charybdotoxin-sensitive K channel by cGMP-dependent protein kinase. Proc. Natl. Acad. Sci. USA 91: 7583–7587.*

Arencibia, J.M., Pastor-Flores, D., Bauer, A.F., Schulze, J.O., Biondi, R.M. (2013). *AGC protein kinases: from structural mechanisms of regulation to allosteric drug development for the treatment of human diseases. Biochim. Biophys. Acta – Proteins and Proteomics 1834: 1302–1321.*

Bahre, H., Hartwig, C., Munder, A., Wolter, S., Stelzer, T., Schirmer, B., Beckert, U., Frank, D.W., Tummler, B., Kaever, V., Seifert, R. (2015). *cGMP and cUMP occur in vivo. Biochem. Biophys. Res. Commun. 460: 909–914.*

Barzik, M., Kotova, T.I., Higgs, H.N., Hazelwood, L., Hanein, D., Gertler, F.B., Schafer, D.A. (2005). Ena/VASP proteins enhance actin polymerization in the presence of barbed end capping proteins. J. Biol. Chem. 280: 28653–28662.

Bear, J.E., Svitkina, T.M., Krause, M., Schafer, D.A., Loureiro, J.J., Strasser, G.A., Maly, I.V., Chaga, O.Y., Cooper, J.A., Borisy, G.G., Gertler, F.B. (2002). Antagonism between Ena/VASP proteins and actin filament capping regulates fibroblast motility. Cell 109: 509–521.

Becker, E.M., Alonso-Alija, C., Apeler, H., Gerzer, R., Minuth, T., Pleib, U., Schmidt, P., Schramm, M., Schroder, H., Schroeder, W., Steinke, W., Straub, A., Stasch, J-P. (2001). NO-independent regulatory site of direct sGC stimulators like YC-1 and BAY 41-2272. BMC Pharmacol. 1: 13–24.

Besant, P.G., Tan, E., Attwood, P.V. (2003). Mammalian protein histidine kinases. Int. J. Biochem. Cell Biol. 35: 297–309; doi:10.1016/S1357-2725(02)00257-1.

Beste, K.Y., Seifert, R. (2013). cCMP, cUMP, cTMP, cIMP and cXMP as possible second messengers: development of a hypothesis based on studies with soluble guanylyl cyclase $\alpha(1)\beta(1)$. Biol. Chem. 394: 261–270.

Blume, C., Benz, P.M., Walter, U., Ha, J., Kemp, B.E., Renne, T. (2007). AMP activated protein kinase impairs endothelial actin cytoskeleton assembly by phosphorylating vasodilator-stimulated phosphoprotein. J. Biol. Chem. 282: 4601–4612.

Breitsprecher, D., Kiesewetter, A.K., Linkner, J., Urbanke, C., Resch, G.P., Small, J.V., Faix, J. (2008). Clustering of VASP actively drives processive, WH2 domain-mediated actin filament elongation. EMBO J. 27: 2943–2954.

Briganti, A., Salonia, A., Gallina, A., Saccà, A., Montorsi, P., Rigatti, P., & Montorsi, F. (2005). Drug insight: oral phosphodiesterase type 5 inhibitors for erectile dysfunction. Nature Clin. Prac. Urology 2: 239–247.

Butt, E., Abel, K., Krieger, M., Palm, D., Hoppe, V., Hoppe, J., Walter, U. (1994). cAMP- and cGMP-dependent protein kinase phosphorylation sites of the focal adhesion vasodilator-stimulated phosphoprotein (VASP) in vitro and in intact human platelets. J. Biol. Chem. 269: 14509–14517.

Chai, S., Chai, Q., Danielsen, C.C., Hjorth, P., Nyengaard, J.R., Ledet, T., Yamaguchi, Y., Rasmussen, L.M., Wogensen, L. (2005). Overexpression of hyaluronan in the tunica media promotes the development of atherosclerosis. Circ. Res. 96: 583–591.

Chamorro-Jorganes, A., Calleros, L., Griera, M., Saura, M., Luengo, A., Rodriguez-Puyol, D., Rodriguez-Puyol, M. (2011). Fibronectin upregulates cGMP-dependent protein kinase type Ibeta through C/EBP transcription factor activation in contractile cells. Am. J. Phys. Cell Phys. 300: C683–691.

Chen, L., Daum, G., Chitaley, K., Coats, S.A., Bowen-Pope, D.F., Eigenthaler, M., Thumati, N.R., Walter, U., Clowes, A.W. (2004). Vasodilator-stimulated phosphoprotein regulates proliferation and growth inhibition by nitric oxide in vascular smooth muscle cells. Arterioscler. Thromb. Vasc. Biol. 24: 1403–1408.

Chen, Z., Zhang, X., Ying, L., Dou, D., Li, Y., Bai, Y., Liu, J., Liu, L., Feng, H., Yu, X., Leung, S.W., Vanhoutte, P.M., Gao, Y. (2014). cIMP synthesized by sGC as a mediator of hypoxic contraction of coronary arteries. Am. J. Physiol. Heart Circ. Physiol. 307: H328–336.

Cheng, A.M., Rizzo-DeLeon, N., Wilson, C.L., Lee, W.J., Tateya, S., Clowes, A.W., Schwartz, M.W., Kim, F. (2014). Vasodilator-stimulated phosphoprotein protects against vascular inflammation and insulin resistance. Am. J. Physiol. Endocrinol. Metab. 307: E571–E579.

Chitaley, K., Chen, L., Galler, A., Walter, U., Daum, G., Clowes, A.W. (2004). Vasodilator-stimulated phosphoprotein is a substrate for protein kinase C. FEBS Lett. 556: 211–215.

Christensen, B., Schack, L., Klaning, E., Sorensen, E.S. (2010). Osteopontin is cleaved at multiple sites close to its integrin-binding motifs in milk and is a novel substrate for plasmin and cathepsin D. J. Biol. Chem. 285: 7929–7937.

Cohen, P. (2002). Protein kinases – the major drug target of the twenty-first century? Nat. Rev. 1: 309–315.

Cornwell, T.L., Lincoln, T.M. (1989). Regulation of intracellular Ca2+ levels in cultured vascular smooth muscle cells: reduction of Ca2+ by atriopeptin and 8-bromo-cGMP is mediated by cGMP-dependent protein kinase. J. Biol. Chem. 264:1146–1155.

Crowther, M.A. (2005). Pathogenesis of atherosclerosis. Hematology Am. Soc. Hematol. Educ. Program 2005: 436–441, doi: 10.1182/asheducation-2005.1.436.

Davidson, J.M., Zoia, O., Liu, J.M. (1993). Modulation of transforming growth factor-beta 1 stimulated elastin and collagen production and proliferation in porcine vascular smooth muscle cells and skin fibroblasts by basic fibroblast growth factor, transforming growth factor-alpha, and insulin-like growth factor-I. J. Cell Physiol. 155: 149–156.

Davies, P.F., Robotewskyj, A., Griem, M.L., Dull, R.O., Polacek, D.C. (1992). Hemodynamic forces and vascular cell communication in arteries. Arch. Path. Lab. Med. 116:1301–1306.

Davis, C.A., Haberland, M., Arnold, M.A., Sutherland, L.B., McDonald, O.G., Richardson, J.A., Childs, G., Harris, S., Owens, G.K., Olson, E.N. (2006). PRISM/PRDM6, a transcriptional repressor that promotes the proliferative gene program in smooth muscle cells. Mol. Cell Biol. 26:2626–2636.

Davis, K.L., Martin, E., Turko, I.V., Murad, F. (2001). Novel effects of nitric oxide. Annu. Rev. Pharmacol. Toxicol. 41: 203–36.

Davis, G.E., Senger, D.R. (2005) Endothelial extracellular matrix biosynthesis, remodeling, and functions during vascular morphogenesis and neovessel stabilization. Circ. Res. 97:1093–1107

Desch, M., Schinner, E., Kees, F., Hofmann, F., Seifert, R., Schlossmann, J. (2010). Cyclic cytidine 3´,5´-monosphosphate (cCMP) signals via cGMP kinase I. FEBS Lett. 584: 3979–3984.

Dey, N.B., Lincoln, T.M. (2012). Possible involvement of cyclic-GMP-dependent protein kinase on matrix metalloproteinase-2 expression in rat aortic smooth muscle cells. Mol. Cell. Biochem. 368: 27–35.

Ding, Q., Chai, H., Mahmood, N., Tsao, J., Mochly-Rosen, D., Zhou, W. (2011). Matrix metalloproteinases modulated by protein kinase Cepsilon mediate resistin-induced migration of human coronary artery smooth muscle cells. J. Vasc. Surg. 53: 1044–1051.

Dollery, C.M., Libby, P. (2006). Atherosclerosis and proteinase activation. Cardiovasc. Res. 69: 625–635.

Doppler, H.R., Bastea, L.I., Lewis-Tuffin, L.J., Anastasiadis, P.Z., Storz, P. (2013). Protein kinase D1-mediated phosphorylations regulate vasodilator-stimulated phosphoprotein (VASP) localization and cell migration. J. Biol. Chem. 288: 24382–24393.

Dubey, R.K., Fingerle, J., Gillespie, D.G., M., Z., Rosselli, M., Imthurn, B., Jackson, E.K. (2015) Adenosine attenuates human coronary artery smooth muscle cell proliferation by inhibiting multiple signaling pathways that converge on cyclin D. Hypertension; doi:10.1161/HYPERTENSIONAHA.115.05912 (in press).

Evanko, S.P., Angello, J.C., Wight, T.N. (1999). Formation of hyaluronan- and versican-rich pericellular matrix is required for proliferation and migration of vascular smooth muscle cells. Arterioscler. Thromb. Vasc. Biol. 19: 1004–1013.

Falk, E. (2006). Pathogenesis of atherosclerosis. J. Am. Coll. Cardiol. 47: C7-C12, doi:10.1016/j.jacc.2005.09.068

Francis, S.H., Corbin, J.D. (1994). Structure and function of cyclic nucleotide-dependent protein kinases. Annu. Rev. Physiol. 56: 237–272.

Fukumoto, S., Nishizawa, Y., Hosoi, M., Koyama, H., Yamakawa, K., Ohno, S., Morii, H. (1997). Protein kinase C delta inhibits the proliferation of vascular smooth muscle cells by suppressing G1 cyclin expression. J. Biol. Chem. 272: 13816–13822.

Gao, Y., Ye, L-H., Kishi, H., Okagaki, T., Samizo, K., Nakamura, A., Kohama, K. (2001). Myosin light chain kinase as a multifunctional regulatory protein of smooth muscle contraction. IUBMB Life 51: 337–344.

Gilotti, A.C., Nimlamool, W., Pugh, R., Slee, J.B., Barthol, T.C., Miller, E.A., Lowe-Krentz, L.J. (2014). Heparin responses in vascular smooth muscle cells involve cGMP-dependent protein kinase (PKG). J. Cell Physiol. 229: 2142–2152.

Gori, T., Parker, J.D. (2002). The puzzle of nitrate tolerance: pieces smaller than we thought? Circulation 106: 2404–2408.

Gomez, D., Owens, G. K. (2012). Smooth muscle cell phenotypic switching in atherosclerosis. Cardiovasc. Res. 95: 156–164.

Hao, H., Ropraz, P., Verin, V., Camenzind, E., Geinoz, A., Pepper, M.S., Gabbiani, G., Bochaton-Piallat, M.L. (2002). Heterogeneity of smooth muscle cell populations cultured from pig coronary artery. Arterioscler. Thromb. Vasc. Biol. 22; 1093–1099.

Henes, J., Schmit, M.A., Morote-Garcia, J.C., Mirakaj, V., Kohler, D., Glover, L., Eldh, T., Walter, U., Karhausen, J., Colgan, S.P., Rosenberger, P. (2009). Inflammation-associated repression of vasodilator-stimulated phosphoprotein (VASP) reduces alveolar-capillary barrier function during acute lung injury. FASEB J. 23: 4244–4255.

Holt, A.W., Tulis, D.A. (2015). Vascular Smooth Muscle as a Therapeutic Target in Disease Pathology, Muscle Cell & Tissue, Ch. 1, pp. 3–25, Ed. K. Sakuma, InTech Open Access Publishers, ISBN 978-953-51-2156-5; http://www. intechopen.com/books/muscle-cell-and-tissue.

Horowitz, A., Clement-Chomienne, O., Walsh, M.P., Tao, T., Katsuyama, H., Morgan, K.G. (1996). Effects of calponin on force generation by single smooth muscle cells. Am. J. Physiol. 270: H1858-H1863.

Huang, C., Chang, J.S., Xu, Y., Li, Q., Zou, Y.S., Yan, S.F. (2010). Reduction of PKCbetaII activity in smooth muscle cells attenuates acute arterial injury. Atherosclerosis 212: 123–130.

Iyer, R.P., de Castro Bras, L.E., Jin, Y.F., Lindsey, M.L. (2014). Translating Koch's postulates to identify matrix metalloproteinase roles in postmyocardial infarction remodeling: cardiac metalloproteinase actions (CarMA) postulates. Circ. Res. 114: 860–871.

Jackson, Jr., E.B., Mukhopadhyay, S., Tulis, D.A. (2007). Pharmacologic modulators of soluble guanylate cyclase/cyclic guanosine monophosphate in the vascular system – from bench top to bedside. Curr. Vasc. Pharmacol. 5: 1–14.

Jenkins, C., Milsted, A., Doane, K., Meszaros, G., Too, J., Ely, D. (2007) A cell culture model using rat coronary artery adventitial fibroblasts to measure collagen production. BMC Cardiovascular Disorders 7:13.

Joshi, C.N., Martin, D.N., Fox, J.C., Mendelev, N.N., Brown, T.A., Tulis, D.A. (2011). The soluble guanylate cyclase stimulator BAY 41-2272 inhibits vascular smooth muscle growth *through the cAMP-dependent protein kinase and cGMP-dependent protein kinase pathways. J. Pharm. Exp. Ther. 339: 394–402.*

Joshi, C.N., Martin, D.N., Shaver, P., Madamanchi, C., Muller-Borer, B.J, Tulis, D.A. (2012). Control of vascular smooth muscle cell growth by connexin 43. Front. Physiol. 3:220. Doi:10.3389/fphys.2012.00220.

Joshi, C.N., Tulis, D.A. (2015). Connexins and intercellular communication in arterial growth and remodeling. Arch. Physiol. 2:1; http://dx.doi.org/10.7243/2055-0898-2-1.

Keswani, A.N., Peyton, K.J., Durante, W., Schafer, A.I., Tulis, D.A. (2009). The cyclic GMP modulators YC-1 and zaprinast reduce vessel remodeling through anti-proliferative and pro-apoptotic effects. J. Cardiovasc. Pharm. Ther. 14: 116–124.

Khalil, R.A. (2010). Regulation of Vascular Smooth Muscle Function. Morgan and Claypool Life Sciences, Bookshelf ID: NBK54586, PMID: 21634065, doi:10.4199/ C00012ED1V01Y201005ISP007.

Kingsley, K., Huff, J.L., Rust, W.L., Carroll, K., Martinez, A.M., Fitchmun, M., Plopper, GE. (2002). ERK1/2 mediates PDGF-BB stimulated vascular smooth muscle cell proliferation and migration on laminin-5. Biochem. Biophys. Res. Commun. 293: 1000–1006.

Kinsella, M.G., Tran, P.K., Weiser-Evans, M.C., Reidy, M., Majack, R.A., Wight, T.N. (2003). Changes in perlecan expression during vascular injury: role in the inhibition of smooth muscle cell proliferation in the late lesion. Arterioscler. Thromb. Vasc. Biol. 23: 608–614.

Knighton, D.R., Zheng, J.H., Ten Eyck, L.F., Ashford, V.A., Xuong, N.H., Taylor, S.S., Sowadski, J.M. (1991). Crystal structure of the catalytic subunit of cyclic adenosine monophosphate-dependent protein kinase. Science 253: 407–414.

Ko, F.N., Wu, C.C., Kuo, S.C., Lee, F.Y., Teng, C.M. (1994). YC-1, a novel activator of platelet guanylate cyclase. Blood 84: 4226–4233.

Komalavilas, P., Penn, R.B., Flynn, C.R., Thresher, J., Lopes, L.B., Furnish, E.J., Guo, M., Pallero, M.A., Murphy-Ullrich, J.E., Brophy, C.M. (2008). The small heat shock-related protein, HSP20, is a cAMP-dependent protein kinase substrate that is involved in airway smooth muscle relaxation. Am. J. Physiol. Lung Cell Mol. Physiol. 294: L69–L78.

Kompa, A.R., Krum, H. (2014). Protein kinases as cardiovascular therapeutic targets. Lancet 384: 1162–1164.

Koyama, H., Raines, E.W., Bornfeldt, K.E., Roberts, J.M., Ross, R. (1996). Fibrillar collagen inhibits arterial smooth muscle proliferation through regulation of Cdk2 inhibitors. Cell 87: 1069–1078.

Koyama, N., Kinsella, M.G., Wight, T.N., Hedin, U., Clowes, A.W. (1998). Heparan sulfate proteoglycans mediate a potent inhibitory signal for migration of vascular smooth muscle cells. Circ. Res. 83: 305–313.

Krause, M., Bear, J.E., Loureiro, J.J., Gertler, F.B. (2002). The Ena/VASP enigma. J. Cell Sci. 115: 4721–4726.

Kwiatkowski, A.V., Gertler, F.B., Loureiro, J.J. (2003). Function and regulation of Ena/VASP proteins. Trends Cell Biol. 13: 386–392.

Lahiry, P., Torkamani, A., Schork, N.J., Hegele, R.A. (2010). Kinase mutations in human disease: interpreting genotype-phenotype relationships. Nature 11: 60–74.

Lee, M.R., Li, L., Kitazawa, T. (1997). Cyclic GMP causes Ca+2 desensitization in vascular smooth muscle by activating the myosin light chain phosphatase. J. Biol. Chem. 272:5063–5068.

Lee, T.H., Sottile, J., Chiang, H.Y. (2015). Collagen inhibitory peptide R1R2 mediates vascular remodeling by decreasing inflammation and smooth muscle cell activation. PLoS One 10: e0117356.

Leitges, M., Elis, W., Gimborn, K., Huber, M. (2001). Rottlerin-independent attenuation of pervanadate-induced tyrosine phosphorylation events by protein kinase C-delta in hemopoietic cells. Lab Invest. 81: 1087–1095.

Lengfeld, J., Wang, Q., Zohlman, A., Salvarezza, S., Morgan, S., Ren, J., Kato, K., Rodriguez-Boulan, E., Liu, B. (2012). Protein kinase C delta regulates the release of collagen type I from vascular smooth muscle cells via regulation of Cdc42. Mol. Biol. Cell 23: 1955–1963.

Li, L., Rui, X., Liu, T., Xu, G., He, S. (2012). Effect of heparin-derived oligosaccharide on vascular smooth muscle cell proliferation and the signal transduction mechanisms involved. Cardiovascular Drugs Ther. 26: 479–488.

Liang, M., Liang, A., Wang, Y., Jiang, J. & Cheng, J. (2014). Smooth muscle cells from the anastomosed artery are the major precursors for neointima formation in both artery and vein grafts. Basic Res. Cardiol.109: 431–449.

Liu, X.M., Peyton, K.J., Mendelev, N.N., Wang, H., Tulis, D.A., Durante, W. (2009). YC-1 stimulates the expression of gaseous monoxide-generating enzymes in vascular smooth muscle cells. Mol. Pharmacol. 75: 1–10.

Madej, T., Lanczycki, C.J., Zhang, D., Thiessen, P.A., Geer, R.C., Marchler-Bauer, A., Bryant, S.H. (2014). MMDB and VAST+: tracking structural similarities between macromolecular complexes. Nucleic Acids Res. 42: D297–D303.

Manning, G., Whyte, D.B., Martinez, R., Hunter, T., Sudarsanam, S. (2002). The protein kinase complement of the human genome. Science 298: 1912–1934; doi: 10.11.1126/science.1075762.

Mendelev, N.N., Williams, V.S., Tulis, D.A. (2009). Anti-growth properties of BAY 41-2272 in vascular smooth muscle cells. J. Cardiovasc. Pharmacol., 53: 121–131.

Newby, A.C. (2005). Dual role of matrix metalloproteinases (matrixins) in intimal thickening and atherosclerotic plaque rupture. Physiol. Rev. 85: 1–31.

Newby, A.C. (2006). Matrix metalloproteinases regulate migration, proliferation, and death of vascular smooth muscle cells by degrading matrix and non-matrix substrates. Cardiovasc. Res. 69: 614–624.

Palumbo, R., Gaetano, C., Melillo, G., Toschi, E., Remuzzi, A., Capogrossi, M.C. (2000). Shear stress downregulation of platelet-derived growth factor receptor-β and matrix metalloprotease-2 is associated with inhibition of smooth muscle cell invasion and migration. Circulation 102: 225–230.

Pearce, L.R., Komander, D., Alessi, D.R. (2010). The nuts and bolts of AGC protein kinases. Nature Rev. Mol. Cell Biol. 11: 9–22.

Rasmussen, H., Takuwa, Y., Park, S. (1987). Protein kinase C in the regulation of smooth muscle contraction. FASEB J. 1: 177–185.

Reffelmann, T., Kloner, R.A. (2003). Therapeutic potential of phosphodiesterase 5 inhibition for cardiovascular disease. Circulation 108: 239–244.

Reinhard, M., Jarchau, T., Walter, U. (2001). Actin-based motility: stop and go with Ena/VASP proteins. Trends Biochem. Sci. 26: 243–249.

Rensen, S.S., Doevendans, P.A., van Eys, G.J. (2007). Regulation and characteristics of vascular smooth muscle cell phenotypic diversity. Neth. Heart J. 15; 100–108.

Rohwedder, I., Montanez, E., Beckmann, K., Bengtsson, E., Duner, P., Nilsson, J., Soehnlein, O., Fassler, R. (2012). Plasma fibronectin deficiency impedes atherosclerosis progression and fibrous cap formation. EMBO Mol. Med. 4: 564–576.

Ross, R. (1993). The pathogenesis of atherosclerosis: a perspective for the 1990s. Nature. 362:801–809.

Ross, R. Glomset, J.A. (1973). Atherosclerosis and the arterial smooth muscle cell. Science. 180: 1332–1339.

Ryer, E.J., Hom, R.P., Sakakibara, K., Nakayama, K.I., Nakayama, K., Faries, P.L., Liu, B., Kent, K.C. (2006). PKCdelta is necessary for Smad3 expression and transforming growth factor beta-induced fibronectin synthesis in vascular smooth muscle cells. Arterioscler. Thromb. Vasc. Biol. 26: 780–786.

Saltore, S., Chiavegato, A., Faggin, E., Franch, R., Puato, M., Ausoni, S., Pauletto, P. (2001) Contribution of adventitial fibroblasts to neointima formation and vascular remodeling from innocent bystander to active participant. Circ Res. 89:1111–1121.

Shi, F., Long, X., Hendershot, A., Miano, J.M., Sottile, J. (2014). Fibronectin matrix polymerization regulates smooth muscle cell phenotype through a Rac1 dependent mechanism. PLoS One 9: e94988.

Stasch, J.P., Becker, E.M., Alonso-Alija, C., Apeler, H., Dembowsky, K., Feurer, A., Gerzer,, R., Minuth, T., Perzborn, E., Pleib, U., Schroder, H., Schroeder, W., Stahl, E., Steinke, W., Straub, A., Schramm, M. (2001). NO-independent regulatory site on soluble guanylate cyclase. Nature 410: 212–215.

Steffensen, B., Wallon, U.M., Overall, C.M. (1995). Extracellular matrix binding properties of recombinant fibronectin type II-like modules of human 72-kDa gelatinase/type IV collagenase. High affinity binding to native type I collagen but not native type IV collagen. J. Biol. Chem. 270; 11555–11566.

Stone, J.D., Holt, A.W., Vuncannon, J.R., Tulis, D.A. (2015). AMP-activated protein kinase inhibits transforming growth factor-β-mediated vascular smooth muscle cell growth: Implications for a Smad-3-dependent mechanism. Am. J. Physiol. Heart Circ. Physiol. (in press); doi:10.1152/ajpheart.00846.2014.

Stone, J.D., Narine, A., Shaver, P.R., Fox, J.C., Vuncannon, J.R., Tulis, D.A. (2013). AMP-activated protein kinase inhibits vascular smooth muscle cell proliferation and migration and vascular remodeling following injury. Am. J. Physiol. Heart Circ. Physiol. 304: H369–H381.

Stone, J.D., Narine, A., Tulis, D.A. (2012). Inhibition of vascular smooth muscle growth via signaling crosstalk between AMP-activated protein kinase and cAMP-dependent protein kinase. Front. Physiol. 3: 409. doi: 10.3389/fphys.2012. 00409.

Surks, H.K. (2007). cGMP-dependent protein kinase I and smooth muscle relaxation: a tale of two isoforms. Circ. Res. 101: 1078–1080.

Tanindi, A., Sahinarslan, A., Elbeg, S., Cemri, M. (2011). Relationship between MMP-1, MMP-9, TIMP-1, IL-6 and risk factors, clinical presentation, extent and severity of atherosclerotic coronary artery disease. Open Cardiovasc. Med. 5: 110–116.

Terrin, A., Monterisi, S., Stangherlin, A., Zoccarato, A., Koschinski, A., Surdo, N.C., Mongillo, M., Sawa, A., Jordanides, N.E., Mountford, J.C., Zaccolo, M. (2012). PKA and PDE4D3 anchoring to AKAP9 provides distinct regulation of cAMP signals at the centrosome. J. Cell Biol. 198: 607–621.

Thomas, W.A., Florentin, R.A., Reiner, J.M., Lee, W.M., Lee, K.T. (1976). Alterations in population dynamics of arterial smooth muscle cells during atherogenesis. IV. Evidence for *a polyclonal origin of hypercholesterolemic diet-induced atherosclerotic lesions in young swine. Exp. Mol. Pathol. 24:244–260.*

Thomson, D.M., Ascione, M.P., Grange, J., Nelson, C., Hansen, M.D. (2011). *Phosphorylation of VASP by AMPK alters actin binding and occurs at a novel site. Biochem. Biophys. Res. Commun. 414: 215–219.*

Thyberg, J., Hultgardh-Nilsson, A. (1994). *Fibronectin and the basement membrane components laminin and collagen type IV influence the phenotypic properties of subcultured rat aortic smooth muscle cells differently. Cell Tissue Res. 276: 263–271.*

Tran, P.K., Tran-Lundmark, K., Soininen, R., Tryggvason, K., Thyberg, J., Hedin, U. (2004). *Increased intimal hyperplasia and smooth muscle cell proliferation in transgenic mice with heparan sulfate-deficient perlecan. Circ. Res. 94: 550–558.*

Tulis, D.A. (2015). *Novel Cyclic Nucleotide Signals in the Control of Pathologic Vascular Smooth Muscle Growth, Cardiovascular Disease II, Ch. 9, pp. 175–200, iCONCEPT Press, Ltd., ISBN 978-1-922227-560; https://www.iconceptpress. com/books/042-2-1/cardiovascular-disease-ii/.*

Tulis, D.A. (2008). *Novel therapies for cyclic GMP control of vascular smooth muscle growth. Am. J. Ther. 15: 551–564.*

Tulis, D.A. (2004). *Salutary properties of YC-1 in the cardiovascular and hematological systems. Curr. Med. Chem. 2: 343–359.*

Tulis, D.A., Bohl Masters, K.S., Lipke, E.A., Schiesser, R.L., Evans, A.J., Peyton, K.J., Durante, W., West, J.L., Schafer, A.I. (2002). *YC-1-mediated vascular protection through inhibition of smooth muscle cell proliferation and platelet function. Biochem. Biophys. Res. Comm. 291: 1014–1021.*

Tulis, D.A., Durante, W., Peyton, K.J., Chapman, G.B., Evans, A.J., Schafer, A.I. (2000). *YC-1, a benzyl indazole derivative, stimulates vascular cGMP and inhibits neointima formation. Biochem. Biophys. Res. Comm. 279: 646–652.*

Ubersax, J.A., Ferrell, J.E. (2007). *Mechanisms of specificity in protein phosphorylation. Nature Rev. Mol. Cell Biol. 8: 530–541.*

Vigetti, D., Clerici, M., Deleonibus, S., Karousou, E., Viola, M., Moretto, P., Heldin, P., Hascall, V.C., De Luca, G., Passi, A. (2011). *Hyaluronan synthesis is inhibited by adenosine monophosphate-activated protein kinase through the regulation of HAS2 activity in human aortic smooth muscle cells. J. Biol. Chem. 286: 7917–7924.*

Walsh, M.P., Horowitz, A., Clement-Chomienne, O., Andrea, J.E., Allen, B.G., Morgan, K.G. (1996). *Protein kinase C mediation of Ca(2+)-independent contractions of vascular smooth muscle. Biochem. Cell Biol. 74: 485–502.*

Wang, S., Song, P., Zou, M-H. (2012). AMP-activated protein kinase, stress response and cardiovascular disease. Clin. Sci. (London) 122: 555–573.

Wang, W.L., Yeh, Y.T., Chen, L.J., Chiu, J.J. (2014). Regulation of fibrillar collagen-mediated smooth muscle cell proliferation in response to chemical stimuli by telomere reverse transcriptase through c-Myc. Biomaterials 35: 3829–3839.

Webb, R.C. (2003). Smooth muscle contraction and relaxation. Adv. Physiol. Educ. 27: 201–206.

Welser, J.V. (2007) Regulation of Smooth Muscle Cell Phenotype by the Alpha7beta1 Integrin. University of Nevada, Reno. https://books.google.com/books?id=guXcVl8NFHYC

White, C.R., Frangos, J.A. (2007). The shear stress of it all: the cell membrane and mechanochemical transduction. Phil. Trans. Royal Soc. Lond. Series B Biol. Sci. 362: 1459–1467.

Woodrum, D., Pipkin, W., Tessier, D., Komalavilas, P., Brophy, C.M. (2003). Phosphorylation of the heat shock-related protein, HSP20, mediates cyclic nucleotide-dependent relaxation. J. Vasc. Surg. 37: 874–881.

World Health Organization; World Heart Federation; World Stroke Organization. (2011). Global atlas on cardiovascular disease prevention and control: Policies, strategies and interventions. ISBN: 978 92 4 156437 3.

Worner, R., Lukowski, R., Hofmann, F., Wegener, J.W. (2007). cGMP signals mainly through cAMP kinase in permeabilized murine aorta. Am. J. Physiol. Heart Circ. Physiol., 292: H237–H244.

Wu, C.C., Ko, F.N., Kuo, S.C., Lee, F.Y., Teng, C.M. (1995). YC-1 inhibited human platelet aggregation through NO-independent activation of soluble guanylate cyclase. Br. J. Pharmacol. 116: 1973–1978.

Yin, X., Bern, M., Xing, Q., Ho, J., Viner, R., Mayr, M. (2013) Glycoproteomic analysis of the secretome of human endothelial cells. Mol Cell Proteomics. 12: 956–978.

Chapter 3

Rhabdomyolysis after Concomitant Use of Statins and Antibiotics

Maria Paparoupa[1] ,Huy Ho[2], Adrian Gillissen[3]

1   Introduction

Acute rhabdomyolysis is defined as a condition of skeletal muscle cell damage leading to release of intracellular materials into the blood stream, such as creatine kinase (CK), myoglobin, uric acid, calcium, phosphate and potassium. Although consensus criteria for rhabdomyolysis is lacking, a reasonable definition is elevation of serum creatine kinase activity of at least 10 times the upper limit of normal followed by a rapid decrease of the sCK level to (near) normal values (Zutt *et al.*, 2014). This clinical and laboratory syndrome typically presents with the triad of myalgia, muscle weakness, and urin darkness, but sometimes rhabdomyolysis can be totally asymptomatic. The diagnosis is based on the elevated creatine kinase levels in serum after exclusion of myocardial infarction. More often comes to myoglobinuria and elevated potassium levels in serum. Some of the muscle damage products such as myoglobin can be harmful for the kidney function, leading to acute renal injury (AKI) or in more severe cases to acute renal failure with elevation of renal retention parameters and need of hemodialysis (Petejova & Martinek, 2014). Rhabdomyolysis can be life-threatening when it comes to acute renal failure, compartment syndrome or cardiac abnormalities (Khan, 2009).

[1] Intensive Care Unit, Klinikum Kassel, University Hospital of Southampton, Germany

[2] Department of Gastroenterology, Klinikum Kassel, University Hospital of Southampton, Germany

[3] Department of Pulmonary Medicine, Klinikum Kassel, University Hospital of Southampton, Germany

Acute rhabdomyolysis can occur under a wide range of disorders like mechanical or heat injury, exposition to poisonous compounds, viruses like *Influenza A and B virus, Parainfluenza typ 1 and 2 virus, Coxcackie virus, HIV 1-2 virus*, endocrinological abnormalities, autoimmunmyositis and drugs (Efstratiadis *et al.*, 2007). Although initially described to be induced by crush injury or trauma, more common causes in hospitalized patients include co-administration of interacting drug agents (Zimmerman & Shen, 2013). The identification of a drug-induced rhabdomyolysis is important because the adverse effect is usually reversible after withdrawal of the suspected compound (Tangiisuran *et al.*, 2009).

Particularly HMG-CoA reductase inhibitors or statins are well-known for their myotoxic potential especially in genetic susceptible individuals (Needham & Mastaglia, 2014). The severity of the myotoxic effect varies from myalgia (2 to 11%) to myositis (0.5%) and rhabdomyolysis (0.1%) (Tomaszewski *et al.*, 2011). Rhabdomyolysis caused by statins can become life-threatening when acute renal failure (ARF) or drug induced liver injury (DILI) occurs. Despite their widespread use, the HMG-CoA reductase inhibitors are an uncommon cause of idiosyncratic DILI. Recent studies have shown that statins are actually safe and efficacious to use in hyperlipidemic patients with chronic liver disease (Rangnekar & Fontana, 2011). Multiple mechanisms of DILI have been implicated, including TNF-alpha-activated apoptosis, inhibition of mitochondrial function and neoantigen formation. Risk factors for DILI include age, sex and genetic polymorphisms of drug-metabolising enzymes such as cytochrome P450 (Hussaini & Farrington, 2007).

Rhabdomyolysis due to statins is mainly observed at the beginning of the treatment, after changing the agent (Khanna & Mundell, 2011), or even after increasing the dose of the subscribed medication (Tayal & Carroll, 2013). The mean onset of myopathy side effects is approximately 6 months after initiation of treatment, but symptoms can occur at any time during the statin therapy (Hansen *et al.*, 2005). Although the risk of rhabdomyolysis is uncommon under a statin therapy alone, it substantially increases in concurrent therapy with inhibitors of cytochrome P450 3A4, which is the main statins `metabolizing liver enzyme. Pharmacologic agents that are also metabolized via this pathway may interact with statins and cause rhabdomyolysis. The risk of statin-induced rhabdomyolysis is increased significantly when statins are used concomitantly with such drugs as fibrates, cyclosporine, macrolide antibiotics, and azole antifungals (Omar *et al.*, 2001). More common interactions can occur between statins and antibiotics, as both medications are frequently co-administered in hospitalized and ambulatory patients. The current review intends to provide an insight of reported interactions between statins and antibacterial agents leading to rhabdomyolysis and elucidate the pathophysiological mechanisms to be involved. Reported interactions between statins and antiviral or antifugal agents will be not included to this text.

2   Methods

Relevant clinical literature was accessed using PubMed (February 1991 – July 2014). The following MESH terms were used: rhabdomyolysis, statins, HMG-CoA reductase inhibitors, antibiotics, adverse events, macrolide.

3   Most Common Interactions

The most common interaction to be reported is between statins and macrolides. The first publication describing the adverse event of rhabdomyolysis after co-administration of simvastatin and clarithromycin appears in 2001 from Lee AJ and Maddix DS (Lee & Maddix, 2001). Several years after the description of the first case, two more macrolides, erythromycin (Molden & Andersson, 2007) and azithromycin (Alreja *et al.*, 2012) are reported to accelerate the myotoxic effect of concomitant prescribed simvastatin. Cases of life-threatening rhabdomyolysis after macrolides (in this case erythromycin) and simvastatin concomitant use can be found in the literature (Fallah *et al.*, 2013). Macrolide antibiotics can lead to myotoxicity without concurrent use of other medications (Brener *et al.*, 2009) and this side effect confuses the evaluation of drug-drug interaction cases.

Reported cases of rhabdomyolysis after co-prescription of macrolides with other groups of statins appear even earlier in the literature. On 1991, Spach *et al.*, (1991) give the first description of an interaction between lovastatin and erythromycin and 1997 two more cases of lovastatin-induced rhabdomyolysis possibly associated with clarithromycin and azithromycin are provided by Grunden and Fisher (1997).

Another antibiotic group reported to induce rhabdomyolysis when subscribed in combination with simvastatin are fluoroquinolones, with ciprofloxacin (Sawant, 2009) and levofloxacin (Paparoupa *et al.*, 2014) as representatives of this category. A well-known interaction exists between fusidic acid and simvastatin (Burtenshaw *et al.*, 2008; Yuen & McGarity, 2003) or fusidic acid and atorvastatin (O'Mahony *et al.*, 2008; Wenisch *et al.*, 2000). Even amoxicillin can cause rhabdomyolysis when co-administrated with simvastatin (Bhatia, 2004).

In all reported cases statins were included to the patient's former medication for at least 6 months and were in the rule well tolerable till antibiotics were initiated. Rhabdomyolysis occurs after prescription of antibiotics with mean interval of 13 days, a minimum of 5 days and a maximum of 4 weeks (Table 1).

Rhabdomyolysis is in most of the cases reversible after discontinuation of suspected medication and acute renal failure occurs occasionally, mainly in patients with already impaired renal function, such as elderly or individuals with chronic renal dysfunction (Table 2). A particular sex predisposition doesn't seem to be relevant referring to appearance of the syndrome or development of severe complications.

Statins, on the other hand, can have a positive effect when combined with antibiotics. Statins and macrolides have a broad immunomodulatory activity and their impact, separately and together, on the survival of patients with sepsis have been evaluated. Patients having statins in the former medication at the time of their admission due to pneumococcal pneumonia were found to have a better clinical outcome, in comparison with those who had not. On the other hand, treatment with a macrolide alone or in combination with statins in this group did not appear to provide a survival benefit

Statin	Antibiotic	Complication	Duration Statin Therapy	Duration Antibiotics
Simvastatin	Clarithromycin	Rhabdomyolysis Acute renal failure	6 months	3 weeks
Simvastatin	Erythromycin	Rhabdomyolysis	Stable therapy	1 week
Simvastatin	Azithromycin	Rhabdomyolysis Acute renal failure	Stable therapy	1 week
Simvastatin	Ciprofloxacin	Rhabdomyolysis	Stable therapy	5 days
Simvastatin	Levofloxacin	Rhabdomyolysis	Stable therapy	8 days
Simvastatin	Fusidic Acid	Rhabdomyolysis	Stable therapy	4 weeks
Atorvastatin	Clarithromycin	Rhabdomyolysis	Stable therapy	2 days

Table 1: Duration of therapy till rhabdomyolysis occurred.

Statin	Antibiotic	Gender Age	Report
Simvastatin	Clarithromycin	Man 64	Lee & Maddix (2007)
Simvastatin	Erythromycin	Man 83	Molden & Andersson (2007)
Simvastatin	Azithromycin	Man 73	Alreja *et al.* (2012)
Simvastatin	Ciprofloxacin	Woman 77	Sawant (2009)
Simvastatin	Levofloxacin	Man 70	Paparoupa *et al.* (2014)
Simvastatin	Fusidic Acid	Man 63	Burtenshaw *et al.* (2008)
Atorvastatin	Fusidic Acid	Man 74	O'Mahony *et al.* (2008)
Lovastatin	Clarithromycin Azithromycin		Grunden & Fisher (1997)
Lovastatin	Erythromycin		Spach *et al.* (1991)
Simvastatin	Amoxicillin		Bhatia (2004)

Table 2: Reported cases overview

(Doshi *et al.*, 2013). Thus, initiation of statins in patients with severe sepsis has not provided convincing evidence of mortality reduction. More randomized trials are required in order to provide sufficient data, about their positive or negative immunomodulatory effect (Mermis & Simpson, 2012). Research data suggests that the inhibition of the mevalonate pathway by statins may provide a potential therapeutic strategy to prevent Aminoglycoside-induced nephrotoxicity due to renal proximal tubule accumulation (Antoine *et al.*, 2010).

4   More Complex Interactions

More complex interactions between statins and antibiotics appear in the literature, when a third medication is suspected for the development of rhabdomyolysis (Bouquié *et al.*, 2011, Chouhan *et al.*, 2009; Kotanko *et al.*, 2002; Mah Ming & Gill, 2003; Sipe *et al.*, 2003). In most of the cases clarithromycin is the antibiotic agent to be involved and simvastatin or atorvastatin the concomitant HMG-CoA reductase inhibitor. Pharmacokinetic interactions are responsible for this toxicity. The impairment of liver function through enzyme inhibition decreases the liver metabolism, especially in the setting of polypharmacy. The inhibition of P-glycoprotein, which enhances the intracellular level of medical agents, leads to increased intracellular concentration and subsequently to increased toxicity and moderate hepatic and renal excretion. Moreover, a long-term treatment with many of the referred agents causes chronic renal failure which decreases the renal elimination of medication (Table 3).

Type of Statin	Antibiotic	Another Medication	Reported Case
Atorvastatin	Clarithromycin	Esomeprazol	Ann Pharmacother. 2003 Jun; 37(6):808–811
Atorvastatin	Clarithromycin	Lopinavir/ Ritonavir	AIDS Patient Care STDS. 2003 May; 17(5):207–210.
Simvastatin	Fusidic acid	Tacrolimus	Nephron. 2002 Feb; 90(2):234–235.
Simvastatin	Clarithromycin	Amiodarone	Ann Pharmacother. 2005 Oct; 39(10):1760–1761.
Pravastatin	Azithromycin	Colchicine Cyclosporin	J Clin Rheumatol. 2011 Jan; 17(1):28–30.

Table 3: More complex interactions between statins and antibiotics with participation of a third medication.

5   Adverse Events Identification Policy

The co-administration of cytochrome P450 3A4 (CYP3A4) inhibitors with simvastatin or atorvastatin (CYP3A4-metabolised statins) is associated with increased statin exposure and risk of adverse drug reactions. The co-prescription of CYP3A4-metabolised statins and CYP3A4 inhibitors was found to be very common in UK primary care according to General Practice Research Database (Bakhai *et al.*, 2012). This co-prescription suggests the limited appreciation of potential interactions and strategies to inform prescribers and pharmacists are required. A population-based cohort study in Ontario Canada, from 2003 to 2010 showed that co-prescription of clarithromycin or erythromycin (inhibitors of cytochrome P450-3A4) was associated with a higher risk for hospitalization with rhabdomyolysis in statin users older than 65 years, compared with co-prescription of azithromycin (not inhibitor of cytochrome P450-3A4) (Patel *et al.*, 2013). On the other side, a systematic screening of the World Health Organization Adverse Drug Reaction database, VigiBase, in July 2008, highlighted that azithromycin may lead to rhabdomyolysis when co-administrated with the individual statins atorvastatin, lovastatin and simvastatin. The aim was to examine all reports including rhabdomyolysis-azithromycin and statins in VigiBase to assess if the data were suggestive of an interaction. This analysis showed that reviewing spontaneous reports can add information to drug interactions not established previously (Strandell *et al.*, 2009). Both studies highlighted that drug-drug adverse events can be underestimated when assessed according to the scientific literature, because only the most severe hospitalized cases are reported. A new assessment tool based on individual reports coming from primary care physicians should be established, in order to offer a better overview of occurring drug-drug adverse events.

6   Mechanisms of Statins-Antibiotics Interaction

The mechanisms involved to statins-antibiotics interaction are complicated because individual statins are metabolized by different liver enzymes, to differing degrees and in some cases producing active metabolites. Simvastatin is metabolized mainly in the liver by Cytochrome CYP 3A4 and its active metabolite simvastatin acid is metabolized by Cytochrome CYP 2C8 (Neuvonen *et al.*, 2006). The CYP3A family metabolises also lovastatin, atorvastatin and cerivastatin, whereas CYP2C9 metabolises fluvastatin. The agent cerivastatin is also metabolised by CYP2C8. Pravastatin is not significantly metabolised by the CYP system (Figure 1) (Williams & Feely, 2002).

In clinical practice, the risk of a serious interaction causing myopathy is enhanced when statin metabolism is markedly inhibited. This mechanism seems to be involved when antibiotics (clarithromycin and erythromycin), antifungals (itraconazole and ketoconazole) and antiretrovirals (HIV protease inhibitors) are co-administrated with statins with predominately liver elimination (Table 4). Statins with drug interaction profile relative to cytochrome P450-3A4 (simvastatin and atorvastatin) are markedly increased by exposure to cytochrome P450-3A4 inhibitors (Jacobson, 2004).

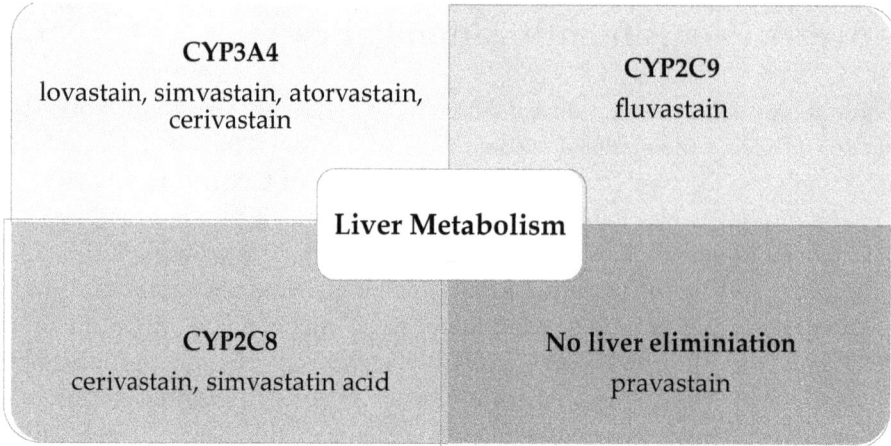

| CYP3A4 | CYP2C9 |
| lovastain, simvastain, atorvastain, cerivastain | fluvastain |

Liver Metabolism

| CYP2C8 | No liver eliminiation |
| cerivastain, simvastatin acid | pravastain |

Figure 1: Lever metabolism of statins.

Statins Metabolised by Cytochrome CYP3A4	Statins Not Metabolised by Cytochrome CYP3A4
Simvastatin	Rosuvastatin
Atorvastatin	Pravastatin
Lovastatin	Fluvastatin
Cerivastatin	
Antibiotics-Antifungals-Antiviral metabolised by Cytochrome CYP3A4	Antibiotics not metabolised by Cytochrome CYP3A4
Clarithromycin	Azithromycin
Erythromycin	Levofloxacin
Itraconazole	Ciprofloxacin
Ketoconazole	
HIV protease inhibitors	

Table 4: HMG-CoA reductase inhibitors and antibiotics categorized according to their metabolism by Cytochrome P450 isoenzyme 3A4 (CYP3A4).

Li *et al.* (2015) conducted a population-based cohort study among older adults taking a statin not metabolized by CYP3A4 (rosuvastatin 76%, pravastatin 21% and fluvastatin 3%) under co-prescription of clarithromycin (metabolized by CYP3A4) versus azithromycin (not metabolized by CYP3A4). The co-prescription of clarithromycin versus azithromycin was associated with a modest but statistically significant increase in the 30-day absolute risk of adverse outcomes (acute kidney injury, admission with hyperkalemia, all-cause mortality) indicated that mechanisms of drug-drug interaction are much more complex than impaired liver elimination.

For instance, statins are substrates of P-glycoprotein (P-gp), also known as MDR1, multiple drug resistance associated proteins (MRPs), which is a cellular drug efflux-transporter responsible for the bioavailability of lots of medications. P-glycoprotein is located in the small intestinal lumen and constitutes a highly efficient barrier for the absorbance of many orally administrated drugs (Pal & Mitra, 2006). The MDR1 system is also responsible for the excretion of liver metabolized drug into the bile. In vitro studies showed that antibiotics with no liver elimination, like levofloxacin, can be a potent inhibitor of P-gp-mediated efflux system. According to this knowledge, levofloxacin for example may have the potential to block the cellular efflux of simvastatin, leading to increased intracellular concentration and subsequent toxicity. The parameter of drug bioavailability becomes more complex as it is strictly connected to lipid or water solubility of a drug and drug metabolites. This characteristic determines the degree of hepatoenteric (lipid solubility) or renal metabolism (water solubility) of the statins.

The human OATP family members OATP1B1 and OATP1B3 (human-organic anion transporting polypeptide (OATP) family) mediate the uptake of endogenous substances and drugs such as antibiotics and HMG-CoA reductase inhibitors (statins) into hepatocytes. OATPs are expressed in a variety of different tissues including brain, intestine, liver, and kidney, suggesting that these uptake transporters are important for drug absorption, distribution, and excretion. Transporter-mediated uptake of drugs into cells determines the drug disposition and is a prerequisite for subsequent liver metabolism.

Seithel *et al.* (2007) investigated the potential role of these uptake transporters on macrolide-induced drug interactions. The macrolides azithromycin, clarithromycin, erythromycin, and roxithromycin inhibited in a concentration-dependent manner the OATP1B1- and OATP1B3-mediated uptake of pravastatin. These results indicate that alterations of uptake transporter function by certain macrolides have to be considered as a potential additional mechanism underlying drug-drug interactions. Because of their wide tissue distribution and broad substrate spectrum, functional consequences of genetic variations (polymorphisms), can contribute to the individual variability of drug effects. Therefore, the molecular characteristics of human OATP family members and genetic variations in SLCO genes encoding OATP proteins should be considered by unexpected drug-drug interactions (König, 2011).

7   Conclusions

Rhabdomyolysis under co-administration of antibiotics and statins is a well demonstrated side effect. Except of well-demonstrated drug-drug interactions, unexpected adverse events may occur. Genetic variations (polymorphisms), can contribute to the individual variability of drug effects. A better overview of occurring drug-drug adverse events can be provided by a reporting system provided by primary care physicians.

References

Alreja, G., Inayatullah, S., Goel, S., Braden, G. (2012). *Rhabdomyolysis caused by an unusual interaction between azithromycin and simvastatin. J Cardiovasc Dis Res. Oct; 3(4):319–22.*

Antoine, D.J., Srivastava, A., Pirmohamed, M., Park, B.K. (2010). *Statins inhibit aminoglycoside accumulation and cytotoxicity to renal proximal tubule cells. Biochem Pharmacol. Feb 15; 79(4):647–54.*

Bakhai, A., Rigney, U., Hollis, S., Emmas, C. (2012). *Co-administration of statins with cytochrome P450 3A4 inhibitors in a UK primary care population. Pharmacoepidemiol Drug Saf. May; 21(5):485–93.*

Bhatia, V. (2004). *Massive rhabdomyolysis with simvastatin precipitated by amoxicillin. J Postgrad Med. Jul–Sep; 50(3):234–5.*

Bouquié, R., Deslandes, G., Renaud, C., Dailly, E., Haloun, A., Jolliet, P. (2011). *Colchicine-induced rhabdomyolysis in a heart/lung transplant patient with concurrent use of cyclosporin, pravastatin, and azithromycin. J Clin Rheumatol. Jan; 17(1):28–30.*

Brener, Z.Z., Bilik, I., Khorets, B., Winchester, J.F., Bergman, M. (2009). *Rhabdomyolysis following clarithromycin monotherapy. Am J Med Sci. Jul; 338(1):78.*

Burtenshaw, A.J., Sellors, G., Downing, R. (2008). *Presumed interaction of fusidic acid with simvastatin. Anaesthesia. Jun; 63(6):656–8.*

Chouhan, U.M., Chakrabarti, S., Millward, L.J. (2005). *Simvastatin interaction with clarithromycin and amiodarone causing myositis. Ann Pharmacother. Oct; 39(10):1760–1.*

Doshi, S.M., Kulkarni, P.A., Liao, J.M., Rueda, A.M., Musher, D.M. (2013). *The impact of statin and macrolide use on early survival in patients with pneumococcal pneumonia. Am J Med Sci. Mar; 345(3):173–7.*

Efstratiadis, G., Voulgaridou, A., Nikiforou, D., Kyventidis, A., Kourkouni, E., Vergoulas, G. (2007). *Rhabdomyolysis updated. Hippokratia. Jul; 11(3):129–37.*

Fallah, A., Deep, M., Smallwood, D., Hughes, P. (2013). *Life-threatening rhabdomyolysis following the interaction of two commonly prescribed medications. Australas Med J. Mar 31; 6(3):112–4.*

Grunden, J.W., Fisher, K.A. (1997). *Lovastatin-induced rhabdomyolysis possibly associated with clarithromycin and azithromycin. Ann Pharmacother. Jul–Aug; 31(7–8):859–63.*

Hansen, K.E., Hildebrand, J.P., Ferguson, E.E., Stein, J.H. (2005). *Arch Intern Med. Dec 12–26; 165(22):2671–6. Outcomes in 45 patients with statin-associated myopathy.*

Hussaini, S.H., Farrington, E.A. (2007). *Idiosyncratic drug-induced liver injury: an overview. Expert Opin Drug Saf. Nov; 6(6):673–84.*

Jacobson, T.A. (2004). *Comparative pharmacokinetic interaction profiles of pravastatin, simvastatin, and atorvastatin when coadministered with cytochrome P450 inhibitors. Am J Cardiol. Nov 1;94(9):1140–6.*

Khan, F.Y. (2009). Rhabdomyolysis: a review of the literature. Neth J Med. Oct; 67(9):272–83.

Khanna, S., Mundell, W.C. (2011). Rhadbomyolysis associated with co-administration of danazol and lovastatin. Br J Clin Pharmacol. Jul; 72(1):166–7.

König, J. (2011). Uptake transporters of the human OATP family: molecular characteristics, substrates, their role in drug-drug interactions, and functional consequences of polymorphisms. Handb Exp Pharmacol; (201):1–28.

Kotanko, P., Kirisits, W., Skrabal, F. (2002). Rhabdomyolysis and acute renal graft impairment in a patient treated with simvastatin, tacrolimus, and fusidic acid. Nephron. Feb; 90(2):234–5.

Lee, A.J., Maddix, D.S. (2001). Rhabdomyolysis secondary to a drug interaction between simvastatin and clarithromycin. Ann Pharmacother. Jan; 35(1):26–31.

Li, D.Q., Kim, R., McArthur, E., Fleet, J.L., Bailey, D.G., Juurlink, D., Shariff, S.Z., Gomes, T., Mamdani, M., Gandhi, S., Dixon, S., Garg, A.X. (2015). Risk of adverse events among older adults following co-prescription of clarithromycin and statins not metabolized by cytochrome P450 3A4. CMAJ. Feb 17; 187(3):174–80.

Mah Ming, J.B., Gill, M.J. (2003). Drug-induced rhabdomyolysis after concomitant use of clarithromycin, atorvastatin, and lopinavir/ritonavir in a patient with HIV. AIDS Patient Care STDS. May; 17(5):207–10.

Mermis, J.D., Simpson, S.Q. (2012). HMG-CoA Reductase Inhibitors for Prevention and Treatment of Severe Sepsis. Curr Infect Dis Rep. Oct; 14(5):484–92.

Molden, E., Andersson, K.S. (2007). Simvastatin-associated rhabdomyolysis after coadministration of macrolide antibiotics in two patients. Pharmacotherapy. Apr; 27(4):603–7.

Needham, M., Mastaglia, F.L. (2014). Statin myotoxicity: A review of genetic susceptibility factors. Neuromuscul Disord. Jan; 24(1):4–15.

Neuvonen, P.J., Niemi, M., Backman, J.T. (2006). Drug interactions with lipid-lowering drugs: mechanisms and clinical relevance. Clin Pharmacol Ther. Dec; 80(6):565–81.

O'Mahony, C., Campbell, V.L., Al-Khayatt, M.S., Brull, D.J. (2008). Rhabdomyolysis with atorvastatin and fusidic acid. Postgrad Med J. Jun; 84(992):325–7.

Omar, M.A., Wilson, J.P., Cox, T.S. (2001). Rhabdomyolysis and HMG-CoA reductase inhibitors. Ann Pharmacother. Sep; 35(9):1096–107.

Pal, D., Mitra, A.K. (2006). MDR- and CYP3A4-mediated drug-drug interactions. J Neuroimmune Pharmacol. Sep; 1(3):323–39.

Paparoupa, M., Pietrzak, S., Gillissen, A. (2014). Acute rhabdomyolysis associated with coadministration of levofloxacin and simvastatin in a patient with normal renal function. Case Rep Med.; 2014: 562929.

Patel, A.M., Shariff, S., Bailey, D.G., Juurlink, D.N., Gandhi, S., Mamdani, M., Gomes, T., Fleet, J., Hwang, Y.J., Garg, A.X. (2013). Statin toxicity from macrolide antibiotic coprescription: a population-based cohort study. Ann Intern Med. Jun 18; 158(12):869–76.

Petejova, N., Martinek, A. (2014). Acute kidney injury due to rhabdomyolysis and renal replacement therapy: a critical review. Crit Care. May 28;18(3):224.

Rangnekar, A.S., Fontana, R.J. (2011). An update on drug induced liver injury. Minerva Gastroenterol Dietol. Jun; 57(2):213–29.

Sawant, R.D. (2009). Rhabdomyolysis due to an uncommon interaction of ciprofloxacin with simvastatin. Can J Clin Pharmacol. Winter; 16(1):e78–9. Epub 2009 Jan 16.

Seithel, A., Eberl, S., Singer, K., Auge, D., Heinkele, G., Wolf, N.B., Dörje, F., Fromm, M.F., König, J. (2007). The influence of macrolide antibiotics on the uptake of organic anions and drugs mediated by OATP1B1 and OATP1B3. Drug Metab Dispos. May; 35(5):779–86.

Sipe, B.E., Jones, R.J., Bokhart, G.H. (2003). Rhabdomyolysis causing AV blockade due to possible atorvastatin, esomeprazole, and clarithromycin interaction. Ann Pharmacother. Jun; 37(6):808–11.

Spach, D.H., Bauwens, J.E., Clark, C.D., Burke, W.G. (1991). Rhabdomyolysis associated with lovastatin and erythromycin use. West J Med. 1991 Feb;154(2):213–5.

Strandell, J., Bate, A., Hägg, S., Edwards, I.R. (2009). Rhabdomyolysis a result of azithromycin and statins: an unrecognized interaction. Br J Clin Pharmacol. 2009 Sep;68(3):427–34.

Tangiisuran, B., Wright, J., Van der Cammen, T., Rajkumar, C. (2009). Adverse drug reactions in elderly: challenges in identification and improving preventative strategies. Age Ageing. 2009 Jul; 38(4):358–9.

Tayal, U. and Carroll, R. (2013). Should anyone still be taking simvastatin 80 mg? BMJ Case Rep. 2013 Aug 8; 2013.

Tomaszwski, M., Stępień, K.M., Tomaszewska, J., Czuczwar, S.J. (2011). Statin-induced myopathies. Pharmacol Rep.; 63(4):859–66.

Wenisch, C, Krause, R, Fladerer, P, El Menjawi, I, Pohanka, E. (2000). Acute rhabdomyolysis after atorvastatin and fusidic acid therapy. Am J Med. 2000 Jul;109(1):78.

Williams, D and Feely, J. (2002). Pharmacokinetic-pharmacodynamic drug interactions with HMG-CoA reductase inhibitors. Clin Pharmacokinet. 2002;41(5):343–70.

Yuen, S.L. and McGarity, B. (2003). Rhabdomyolysis secondary to interaction of fusidic acid and simvastatin. Med J Aust. 2003 Aug 4;179(3):172.

Zimmerman, J.L. and Shen, M.C. (2013). Rhabdomylysis. Chest 2013 Sep; 144(3):1058–65.

Zutt, R., van der Kooi, A.J., Linthorst, G.E., Wanders, R.J., de Visser, M. (2014). Rhabdomyolysis: review of the literature. Neuromuscul Disord. 2014 Aug;24(8):651–9.

Chapter 4

Hemostatic Evaluation of Chitosan Derivatives: Effects on Platelets *In Vitro*

Mercy Halleluyah Periayah[1], Ahmad Sukari Halim[1],
Arman Zaharil Mat Saad[1], Nik Soriani Yaacob[2], Abdul Rahim Hussein[3],
Ahmad Hazri Abdul Rashid[4], Zanariah Ujang[4]

1   Introduction

Since the middle of World War II, half of all recorded combat deaths have occurred as a result of exsanguinating hemorrhage. A military post-mortem study of casualties in Operation Iraqi Freedom suggested that up to 24% of all battlefield mortalities could be eliminated with improved anti-hemorrhaging methods and that 85% of deaths were caused by uncontrolled hemorrhage (Kelly *et al.*, 2008). The development of new methods or devices for hemorrhage control may contribute to a future reduction in hemorrhage morbidity and mortality (Pusateri *et al.*, 2003). In many hospital settings, maintaining a good hemostatic balance in bleeding patients remains a major challenge (Shander, 2007). Successful approaches in hemostasis research may contribute to a significant reduction in hemorrhage related fatalities. Among the novel hemostatic agents approved by the U.S. Food and Drug Administration (FDA), chitosan-based agents have shown great promise in preventing major hemorrhaging in pre-hospital settings and in animal models of major blood loss (Kozen *et al.*, 2008). Recently, a chitosan-derived an-

[1] Reconstructive Sciences Unit, School of Medical Sciences, Universiti Sains Malaysia, Kelantan, Malaysia

[2] Department of Chemical Pathology, School of Medical Sciences, Universiti Sains Malaysia, Kelantan, Malaysia

[3] Advanced Medical & Dental Institute, Universiti Sains Malaysia, Kelantan, Malaysia

[4] Industrial Biotechnology Research Centre, SIRIM Berhad, Selangor, Malaysia

tihemorrhage biomaterial, which contains *N*-acetyl glucosamine (found abundantly as a major component in the shells of arthropods such as crabs, shrimps, lobsters and insects) (Koide *et al.*, 1998), was identified as having potential clinical utility. Chitosan is well known for its potential as a non-toxic, biocompatible and biodegradable product (Jayakumar *et al.*, 2008; Muzzarelli R.A.A; Muzzarelli C., 2009). Chitosan has the ability to expedite the wound healing process and arrest bleeding by facilitating platelet recruitment and promoting coagulation by forming a pseudo-clot. The chitosan structure can be chemically modified and has been widely employed both as a biomaterial scaffold for the controlled release of pharmaceuticals and as a component of successful wound dressing (Khor & Lim, 2001). The compatibility of chitosan biomaterials is a feature of sample preparation, viscosity, molecular weight (MW), degree of deacetylation (DDA), incubation period and temperature. Platelets circulating within the blood are the essential mediators that trigger the mechanical pathway of the coagulation cascade upon encountering any damage to the blood vessels. Driven by the significant role of adherence in the platelet response during the hemostasis process, we have evaluated platelet responses to characterize platelet capacities upon the adherences of chitosan *in vitro*. We predict that varying formulations of chitosan- based hemostatic agents may have different potential roles in expediting hemostasis. In our research, we used *N*,O-Carboxymethylchitosan (NO-CMC) and Oligo-Chitosan (O-C) produced by the Standard and Industrial Research Institute of Malaysia (SIRIM Berhad) with DDA ranging between 75–95%. Lyostypt, a commercial hemostatic agent, was used as a positive control. Additionally, we demonstrated the ability of chitosan-based hemostatic agents to induce platelet and blood coagulation cascades that measure platelet adherences, platelet shape changes, platelet activation, adenosine diphosphate (ADP)-induced platelet aggregation, blood coagulation ability and coagulation profile measurements. We have also successfully reported and published that platelets respond differently to chitosan derivatives with differing MW and DDA (Periayah *et al.*, 2013; 2014). This book chapter aims to provide the extended version of presently published content on chitosan activities towards platelet and blood coagulation mechanisms. Since we are exploring on platelet activities which involve in the coagulation process, as a new contribution to the society, chitosan-based hemostatic agents could be a new strategy biomaterial to achieve hemostasis. Knowledge on various signaling cascades in platelet thrombogenicity is very important in order to develop a novel therapeutic chitosan based treatment for hemorrhage. Since chitosan is a biodegradable biopolymer, it causes no hazard to the environment.

2   Materials and Methods

2.1   Materials

We used NO-CMC and O-C produced by the SIRIM Berhad with a DDA of 75–95%. Chitosan sponges with variable chitosan formulations (7% NO-CMC with 0.45 mL of collagen, 8% NO-CMC, O-C and one powdered type of chitosan termed O-C 53) were used. Lyostypt was used as the positive control.

2.2   Subject Selection

We recruited 14 healthy donors aged 18 to 50 who had not consumed any drugs in the previous two weeks. Informed written consent was obtained prior to the blood collection. None of the women were taking oral contraceptives when the blood samples were obtained. None of the participants had a diagnosis of a chronic disease. Prior to commencing the study, ethical clearance was obtained from the Human Ethics Committee of the Universiti Sains Malaysia (USM) (Ref Num: FWA Reg. No: 00007718; IRB Reg. No 00004494). We have assured that identifying information was not made available to anyone who was not directly involved in the study. The stricter standard was the principle of *anonymity*, which essentially indicates that the participant will remain anonymous throughout the study. All the participating donors' personal details remained confidential.

2.3   Blood Collection

Twelve milliliters of whole blood was drawn from the antecubital vein into 3 vials of ethylenediaminetetraacetic acid (EDTA) tubes for all the studies except for the platelet aggregation, activation and coagulation profile studies. To evaluate these expressions, three-way stop-cocks were used to collect blood under minimal tourniquet pressure, and the first 1 mL of blood withdrawn was discarded. The remainder of each blood sample was aliquot into 3 tubes containing trisodium citrate anticoagulant. The subject selection was contingent on the presence of a hematocrit level between 38 and 45% and a normal platelet count between $150 \times 10^3/\mu L$ and $350 \times 10^3/\mu L$.

2.4   Platelet Count and Morphology Studies

2.4.1   Chitosan Preparation

Chitosan samples, each weighing 5 mg, were dissolved or pre-moistened in 50 μL of (PBS) (pH 7.4) and subjected to incubation at 37 °C for 60 minutes (min) (Wagner *et al.*, 1996; Zhou *et al.*, 2008).

2.4.2   Platelet Count

Blood was collected from healthy donors in BD Vacutainer [K2 *EDTA 3.6 mg (REF 367842)]* tubes. Ten tubes were prepared, and 1 mL of blood was added per tube. The blood was introduced to the prepared chitosan samples. A 200 μL aliquot of blood was transferred from each 1 mL tube of whole blood to single vial plain tubes every 10 and 20 min. The platelet counts obtained were compared with the initial baseline counts. The results were analyzed using a Sysmex XE 5000 Automated Hematology Analyzer of Sysmex Corporation (Kobe, Japan) device. The platelet counts were analyzed using the hydro dynamic focusing method based on fluorescence flow cytometry (Sysmex, 2008; Periayah *et al.*, 2013).

2.4.3   Preparation of Platelet and Erythrocyte for the Morphological Analysis of Chitosan Derivatives

Platelets from healthy donors were isolated by differential centrifugation with $150 \times g$ for 15 min and $900 \times g$ for 5 min at room temperature (Salas, 2000). Five hundred milliliters of isolated platelets was combined with each chitosan sample and incubated for 30 min in 12-well tissue culture plates. Each chitosan biomaterial measuring 5 mm × 5 mm was placed in a 12-well tissue culture plate. Each well was then washed with penicillin-infused phosphate-buffered saline (PBS) for 1 hour (hr), fixed in 100 µL of glutaraldehyde for 1 hr, and then washed with distilled water. Different concentrations of ethanol (30%, 70% and 100%) were added to dehydrate the chitosan biomaterials. Finally, all the samples were dried in an incubator (58 ºC) overnight. Once the biomaterials were completely dried, they were subsequently subjected to sputter-coating with gold using a gold sputter coater (Leica SCD 005, Germany) with the following conditions: vacuum millibar of 5×10^{-2}; current of 20 milliampere (mA); time of 150 seconds (sec). The gold sputtered chitosan biomaterials were examined under scanning electron microscope (SEM) (FEI-QUANTA FEG 450, Netherlands); in particular, their surface and cross-section morphology were examined (Okamoto *et al.*, 2003; Periayah *et al.*, 2013). SEM analysis is one of the robust and established technique which can detect by delivering information on biomaterial surface pattern. A drop of whole blood was placed on each slide, and peripheral blood films were prepared. The slides were stained with a Geimsa stain for 5 min and washed with PBS (pH 6.8) for 15 min. The slides were mounted, and the adhered cells were observed using light microscopy (Nikon Eclipse E200). The images were captured using Mirax Desk Zeiss (Okamoto *et al.*, 2003; Genzen and Miller 2005).

2.5   Platelet Activation

2.5.1   Blood Sample Collection and Preparation

Blood samples were collected as described above using BD Vacutainer 0.109 M (3.2%) trisodium citrate anticoagulant tubes (REF 363083) from healthy donors. The blood samples were centrifuged at $1000 \times g$ for 15 min. The supernatants were harvested upon centrifugation. Five hundred microliters of platelet rich plasma (PRP) was then mixed with each prepared chitosan sample for 30 min (Ritchie *et al.*, 2000; Okamoto *et al.*, 2003; Zhou *et al.*, 2008; Periayah *et al.*, 2014). The levels of P-selectin in the serum upon adhesion to the chitosan were measured using an enzyme-linked immunosorbent assay (ELISA) procedure (Cat. No. CSB-E04708 h), and the test was performed according to the manufacturer's instructions.

2.5.2   Platelet Activation Assay Procedure

One hundred microliters of the prepared standard and samples were loaded into each well, and the plate was covered using adhesive strips. The sample-loaded plate was incubated for 2 hr at 37 °C. One hundred microliters of Biotin-Ab (1X) was loaded once the standards and the samples were completely removed from each well. The plate was incubated for 1 hr at 37 ºC. Next, Biotin-Ab (1×) was added, and each well was aspirated and washed using washing buffer (200 µL) twice for a total of three washes using a multichannel pipette every 2 min. One hundred microliters of Biotin-Av (1×) was added to each well, and the plate was incubated for 1 hr at 37ºC. The aspiration or washing procedures were repeated at least 5 times as described previously. Once the final washing was completed, 90 µL of TMB substrate was added to each well, and the plate was protected from light exposure and incubated for 15 to 30 min. As a final solution to the plate, 50 µL of stop solution was added to the entire well, and the plate was gently tapped to ensure thorough mixing. Eventually, all the reactions were stopped, and the absorbance was determined at 450 nm utilizing an ELISA reader (Tecan Infinite 200 PRO NanoQuant, Switzerland). A standard curve was generated, and the concentration of each sample was determined in ng/mL. The protein expression was calculated based on the volume of supernatant obtained after clot retraction. The standard curve was generated by plotting the absorbance for each standard on the y-axis against its concentration on the x-axis and drawing a 4-parametric logistic curve-fit that was plotted through all the data points (Garbaraviciene *et al.*, 2010). No significant cross-reactivity or interference was observed among all the measurement levels.

2.6   Platelet Aggregation

Blood was collected in BD Vacutainer 0.109 M (3.2%) trisodium citrate anticoagulant tubes (REF 363083) from healthy donors. Platelet aggregation was measured in a Chronolog lumi-aggregometer (Chrono-Log, Havertown, PA) at 37 °C, under stirring. Platelet aggregation was determined by measuring changes in the optical density (i.e., light transmittance) of the stirred chitosan-adhered whole blood after the addition of an aggregating agent to the aggregometer cuvette. Five hundred microliter samples of chitosan-adhered whole blood were diluted in normal saline and pre-warmed for 5 min in the incubation well. The baseline was determined using the platelet suspension diluted 1:1 with a platelet suspension buffer to increase the gain of the aggregometer output. The luminescence gains were decreased to the minimum value by turning the rotary switch to 0.05. The stirring speeds were set to 1200 × *g*. A total of 10 µL of CHRONO-LUME® (ADP) was added to each sample, and the luminescence gain setting was recorded. The peak luminescence or the amplitude was recorded in ohms (Ω). Generally, each platelet aggregation ran for at least 2 min and occasionally up to 5 min. The chart speed of the recorder varies by the type of equipment, but it should be sufficiently fast to observe the change in the shape of the aggregation tracing, which is usually 2 mm or more per min. This amount of time allowed the observation of the first- and second-wave aggregation for ADP (Zhou and Schmaier, 2005; Periayah *et al.*, 2013). The platelet aggregation test was performed within 3 hr of blood collection upon venipuncture to avoid false platelet aggregations.

2.7   Coagulation Profiles Study

2.7.1   Blood Coagulation Study

Two milliliters of blood was drawn from the antecubital vein of each of the healthy donors for a total of 12 mL, which was stored in BD Vacutainer [K2 *EDTA 3.6 mg (REF 367842)*] tubes. To prepare the PRP blood, it was centrifuged at 1200 × *g* for 3 min. Platelet-poor plasma (PPP) was withdrawn from the top of the centrifuged tube using a sterile needle, leaving 1 mL of PRP in each tube. Each type of chitosan was tested in duplicate. The blood samples from each donor that weighed 100 mg were dissolved in 100 μL of PBS (pH 7.4) and incubated at 37 °C for 30 min. After 30 min, 1 mL of whole blood or PRP was added to each of the 1.5 mL Eppendorf tubes. The time at which the blood coagulated was recorded for each chitosan sample, and after 15 min, the tests were stopped (Wagner *et al.*, 1996; Robin *et al.*, 2012; Periayah *et al.*, 2013; 2014). The blood clot formed on each sample was photographed with a digital camera (Fujifilm Finepix J150W, Japan).

2.7.2   Coagulation Factors Analysis

Ten milliliters of blood was collected in BD Vacutainer 0.109 M (3.2%) trisodium citrate anticoagulant tubes (REF 363083). The blood was kept warm and centrifuged at 3000 × *g* for 10 min at 22 °C to obtain platelet poor plasma (PPP). The PPP was prepared in accordance with the approved guidelines of the Clinical and Laboratory Standard Institute. The PPP was briefly agitated on a vortex mixer. Five hundred milliliters of isolated PPP was combined with 10 mg of prepared chitosan that had pre-absorbed 50 μL of PBS; this mixture was incubated for 10 min. The activated partial thromboplastin time (APTT), the prothrombin time (PT), the thrombin time (TT) and fibrinogen (Fib) were measured using a STA Compact Coagulation Analyzer (Diagnostica Stago, France) according to the manufacturer's instructions. Coagulation profiles were evaluated by pre-warming and incubating samples. The samples were calcified automatically in the machine vials and the tests were performed according to the manufacturer's instructions. Plasma was calcified and clotting was initiated by adding the Stago reagents. The quality control measurements were set in the proper range according to standard clinical laboratory protocol prior to testing (Maurer *et al.*, 2001; Arkin *et al.*, 2003; Yang *et al.*, 2007; Periayah *et al.*, 2014).

2.8   Statistical Analysis

We used a repeated-measure analysis of variance (ANOVA) and the correlation coefficient to identify statistical trends for the platelet count test, which was compared using 3 different time intervals. Statistical significance was also compared using a one-way ANOVA, and an independent *t*-test. Statistical significance was defined as $P \leq 0.05$, and these values were calculated using SPSS software, version 20.0. All the quantitative experimental outcomes were elucidated in percentages and means ± standard error of the mean (S.E.M).

3. Results and Discussion

3.1 Assessment and Effects of Platelet Adhesion on the Adherences of Different Types of Chitosan

3.1.1 Platelet Count

Chitosan has become one of the most promising local hemostatic agents. It is of particular importance because it functions independently on platelets and normal clotting mechanisms. This present study was constructed to conduct a platelet adhesion test to illustrate the clear actions of chitosan on platelet counts and its morphology. Platelet counts were tested upon the adherences of chitosan biomaterials at three different time intervals including baseline, after 10 min and after 20 min. The rationale of this analysis was to study the lowest level of platelet counts because as the platelet count is reduced, the chances for the platelets to be attracted to chitosan increase. This measurement identifies materials that may be more effective as hemostatic agents (Periayah *et al.*, 2013).

Previous reports described comparative studies that were performed in a controlled *in vitro* environment that was associated with human blood and plasma. This study was designed to estimate the standard properties of available hemostatic agents. The interactions between the coagulation system and polymer surfaces are highly complex and require the proportional blood compatibility of biomaterials (Saito *et al.*, 1997; Kirkpatrick *et al.*, 1998; Sieminski and Gooch, 2000). Naturally derived polymers have the benefits of biological attributes such as cell proliferation and biocompatibility, and their application is an extension of their biological purpose.

The utilization of controlled *in vitro* techniques as screening tools aids the process of generating novel hemostatic agents. The composition of chitosan is a potential supplementary tool for the investigation of hemostasis (Cheng *et al.*, 2009; Xiangmei *et al.*, 2009). Platelets can adhere to the surfaces of biomaterials. Platelet number counting is an important tool for assessing hemocompatibility because the platelet number influences the formation of a hemostatic plug or thrombus (Bernacca *et al.*, 1998; Turner *et al.*, 2002). The outcome was analyzed using a repeated measure ANOVA test to observe the platelet counts at 3 different time intervals. A repeated measure ANOVA was employed because it is the only statistical design that could be possibly used to obtain information concerning individual patterns of change and repeatedly measure the same variable over time on the same group of subjects.

The platelet counts were observed to decrease significantly ($p < 0.05$) upon the adherences of all the tested chitosan biomaterials except for blood alone. The largest decrease was observed in O-C with the following values: baseline: $303.1 \pm 9.54 \times 10^3/\mu L$; after 10 min: $260.1 \pm 12.6 \times 10^3/\mu L$; and after 20 min: $249.1 \pm 12.7 \times 10^3/\mu L$. The next most prominent decrease was noted in O-C 53 with the following values: baseline: $308.9 \pm 12.2 \times 10^3/\mu L$; after 10 min: $275.5 \pm 10.8 \times 10^3/\mu L$; and after 20 min: $258.4 \times 10^3/\mu L$. The percentage changes in the platelet counts increased from 10.8% (after 10 min) to 16.35% (after 20 min). Subsequently, lyostypt, 7% NO-CMC and 8% NO-CMC recorded 8.7, 5.7 and 4.6% platelet count decreases during the first 10 min of the analysis, respectively. Meanwhile, 13.3, 9.6 and 10% decreases were registered after 20 min by lyostypt, 7% NO-CMC and

8% NO-CMC, respectively (Figure 1). No significant values were observed between the each of the tested biomaterials and the each time period.

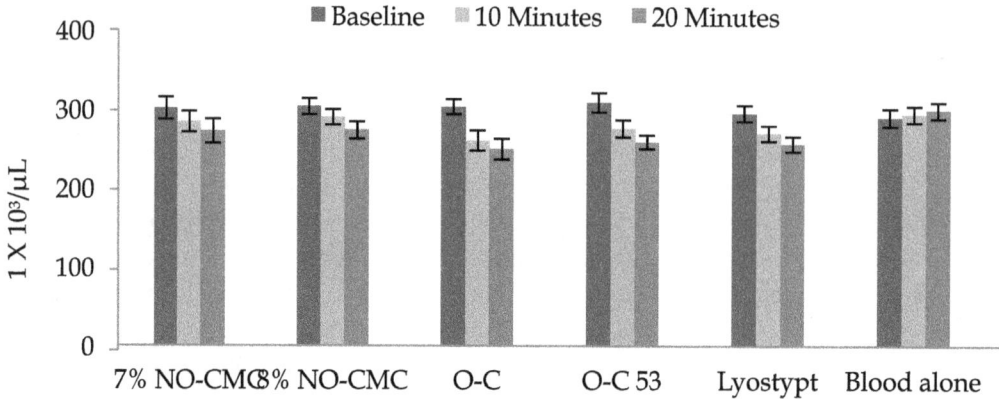

Figure 1: Mean value of platelet counts upon the adherence of chitosan. The error bars indicate the S.E.M. ($n = 14$).

On the other hand, Pearson's correlation was applied to measure the relationships between the 3 different time intervals. Usually, Pearson's correlation is a measure of the strength and direction of a linear relationship between two variables. If the relationship between the variables is not linear, the correlation coefficient will not be able to elucidate the strength of the relationship between the variables (Lane, 2014). The analysis of correlation indicated that the relationship between the baseline, the 10 min interval and the 20 min interval was strong. This positive correlation indicates that for all tested biomaterials, except for blood alone, the platelet counts decreased to a significant degree. The correlation between baseline and 10 min was characterized by $r = 0.83$ and $p < 0.01$. The observed correlation between baseline and 20 min was characterized by $r = 0.73$ and $p < 0.01$. The strongest relationship was noted between 10 and 20 min, which had the value of $r = 0.94$ ($p < 0.01$). Pearson's correlation (r) indicates that the measurements were performed with samples and not with populations. Pearson's r ranges from –1 to 1. An r of –1 indicates a perfect negative linear relationship between variables, an r of 0 indicates no linear relationship between variables, and an r of 1 indicates a perfect positive linear relationship between variables (Periayah *et al.*, 2013).

Lyostypt was used as the positive control. Lyostypt is composed of collagen, which exhibits excellent biocompatibility and has a significant role in primary and secondary hemostasis. Collagen-based chitosan was utilized because collagen has the ability to initiate platelet adherences at the site of bleeding tissues (Seda *et al.*, 2007). Collagens are crucially important for platelet adhesion and subsequent activation on the extracellular matrix of denuded endothelium (Wilner *et al.*, 1971). In this study, 7% NO-CMC chitosan coated with 0.45 mL of ovine collagen was used. The collagen was mixed with NO-CMC in predetermined compositions and freeze-dried to obtain a porous structure. No significant results were observed upon the adherences of the collagen coated NO-CMC in comparison with O-C. This was likely because of the different MW, DDA, functional groups and scaffold porosities of NO-CMC and O-C.

The rapid and accurate determination of platelet counts is a crucial factor in diagnostic pathology. The main reason an automated hematology analyzer was used in this study is that this analyzer is usually capable of providing accurate platelet counts with a generally good precision (Gao *et al.*, 2013). Previously, it has been reported that chitosan is fully capable of stimulating platelet adhesion in a time-dependent manner of within a 5 to 30 min time period (Chou *et al.*, 2003). In this present investigation on platelet quantification, the count tended to decrease upon the adherences of chitosan biomaterials within 2 different time intervals. A greater decrease of platelets resulted in more chitosan biomaterial that was capable of entrapping platelets on the surface membrane. Because platelet adhesion is an essential function in response to vascular injury and is generally viewed as the first step during the coagulation process, this quantification of platelets is useful for elucidating the significant role of chitosan biomaterials on attracting more platelets for the hemostasis process.

3.1.2   Morphological Analysis of Chitosan-Adhered Platelets

Surface membrane properties possess an enormous effect on the biocompatibility action of a biomaterial. Factors such as surface characterization, porosity evaluation, thickness and tensile strengths are the central issues in biomaterial research for correlating with biological performances. The success of using microscopic methods to characterize biomaterial surfaces is well established, and these microscopy techniques were often found in the biomaterials literature (Merrett *et al.*, 2002). SEM and light microscopy have been used to study the morphological changes of the platelets upon the adherence of chitosan biomaterials.

The platelet morphology was observed by SEM. The greatest number of platelet attachments was observed on the tested chitosan biomaterials because nearly 90% of the platelets adhered to the chitosan surface membrane. Most platelets were irregular and pseudopodal in shape.

Figure 2A–2E shows observations of these shapes under different magnifications (8000×, 6000×, 3500×, 500×, and 10000×). These varying shapes are a result of the differing surface properties of the biomaterials. The contact angle of O-C 53 (Figure 2D) under 500× was 200 μM in diameter. Because O-C 53 is a powder, observation at a higher magnification was ineffective because the beam could not readily penetrate the sample to detect platelet contact with the desired crossover diameter and failed to form an acceptable image. The platelets were appeared to have irregular shapes and did not display any granulation. Aggregated platelets had already discharged their granules, as shown in Figure 2A–2C. No single platelets were observed. Platelets clumped to form a large group, forming a fibrin clot that reinforced platelet aggregation. The results showed a positive increase compared to those of lyostypt, which was composed of highly flexible strands that allowed the platelets to form fibrin networks (Figure 2E).

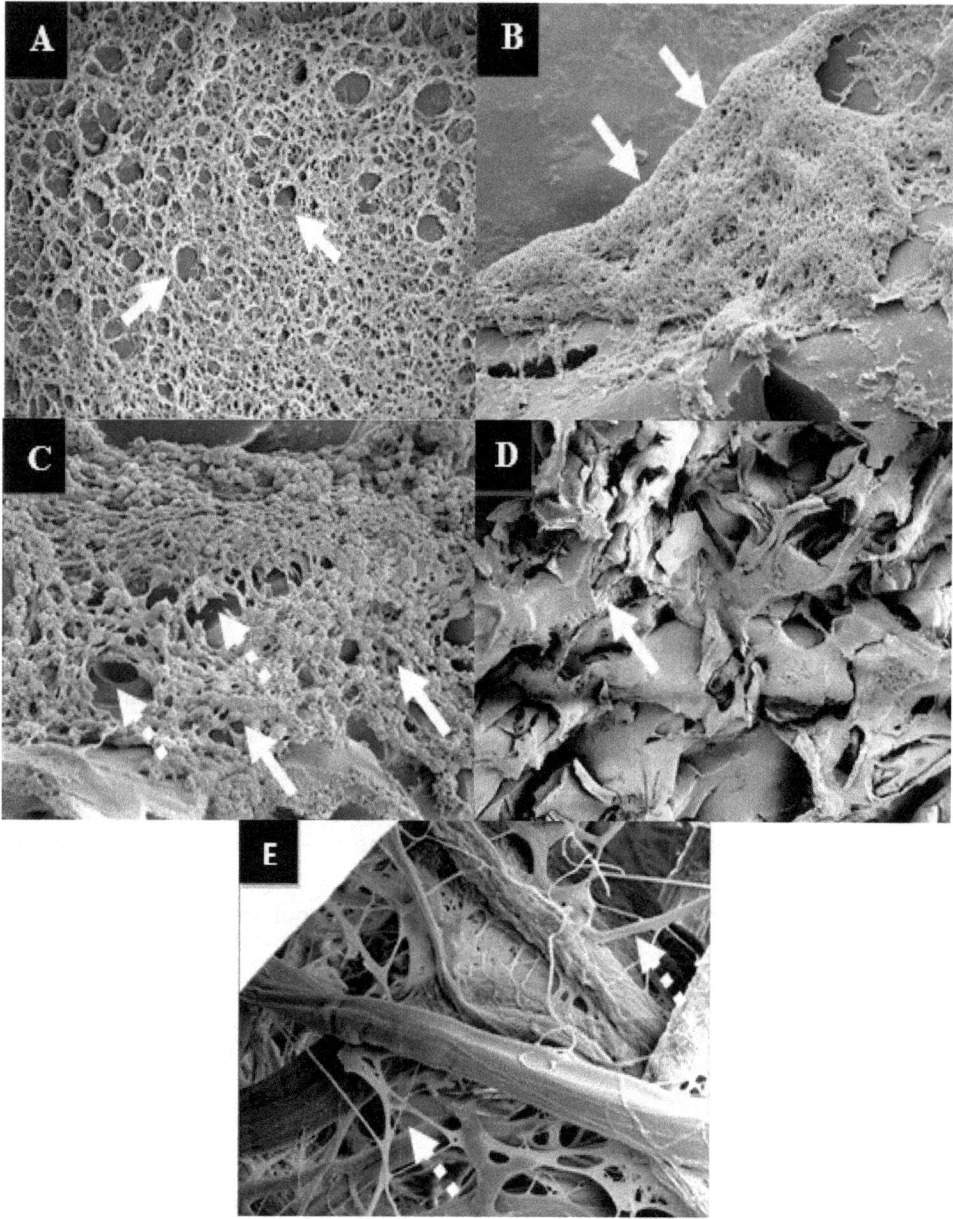

Figure 2: Platelet morphology upon the adherences of NO-CMCs, O-Cs and lyostypt. [(A) 7% NO-CMC. (B) 8% NO-CMC. (C) O-C. (D) O-C 53. (E) Lyostypt]. The platelet shapes changed into irregular pseudopodals upon aggregation (solid white arrow). Fibrin meshes formed upon blood coagulation (dashed white arrow).

The SEM analysis showed that the platelets adhered to one another, clumping into irregular shapes and elongated pseudopod forms, depending on the type of chitosan material. These chitosan materials varied based on their DDA and MW. O-C appeared yellow in color, and the surface of the material was harder than those of the other types of chitosan. This distinction likely appeared because O-C was exposed to slightly higher localized temperatures during the production stage. The platelets formed abnormal shapes and exhibited varying degrees of surface roughness and surface wettability (hydrophilic and hydrophobic surfaces) (Laka and Chernyavskaya, 2006). The shapes of the platelets changed from discoid-shaped resting cells to spiculated spheres. O-C 53 attracted more platelets to form bridges, most likely because the degree of crystallinity of O-C 53 was higher (Kuwahara *et al.*, 2002). The broad, irregular spread of the platelets ensures firm adhesion in an irreversible mode (Periayah *et al.*, 2013; 2014). Upon morphological analysis, platelet attachments were detected on most of the chitosan surfaces. The platelets adhered to one another and extended into pseudopodal forms to aggregate depending on their surface roughness, thickness and absorbability.

Peripheral blood smears were prepared to examine the characteristics of blood cells upon the adherences of the chitosan biomaterials. A Geimsa stain is a classic blood film stain for peripheral blood smears that is normally used to differentiate the nuclear or cytoplasmic morphology of platelets, red blood cells or erythrocytes, white blood cells and parasites. The stains or the morphology of the erythrocytes are stained in pink or red; the platelets in purple or pink; the lymphocytes in light blue; the monocytes in pale blue and the leukocytes in magenta (M15A, NCCLS, 2000; Garcia, 2001). Light microscopy employs visible light to detect tiny objects. It is easy to handle, provides superlative image quality and is cost-efficient. The images of the stained smears were captured using Mirax Desk Zeiss, which is a robust and stable base scanner capable of capturing Geimsa-stained smear slides.

Erythrocyte morphology was assessed by a peripheral blood smear (Figure 3). The clearest finding from this study was that erythrocyte aggregations were observed in all the chitosan-adhered biomaterials. Irregular aggregations of erythrocytes into grape-like clusters and the aggregation of platelet cells were observed in both NO-CMC samples (Figure 3A–3B). Fibrin meshes also formed around the erythrocyte aggregations (Figure 3A, 3E). However, in the presence of both O-Cs, the erythrocytes swelled and aggregated vigorously. Platelet aggregation was difficult to observe because the erythrocytes covered 80% of the chitosan surface (Figure 3C, 3D). Similarly, in the presence of lyostypt, the erythrocytes overlaid maximally, but in this case, the fibrin mesh was clearly visible (Figure 3E). This outcome shows that the adhesion and aggregation of erythrocytes was stimulated and induced by NO-CMC and O-C. The aggregations of erythrocytes and platelets together with the formation of a fibrin meshes in the peripheral blood films were successfully observed. The hydrophilic surface properties of chitosan derivatives promoted platelet adhesion and activation in achieving hemostasis. The purpose of this figure is to express differences between platelet and erythrocyte aggregations which distinguish the shapes and the degree of membrane coverage of the erythrocyte on chitosan biomaterials.

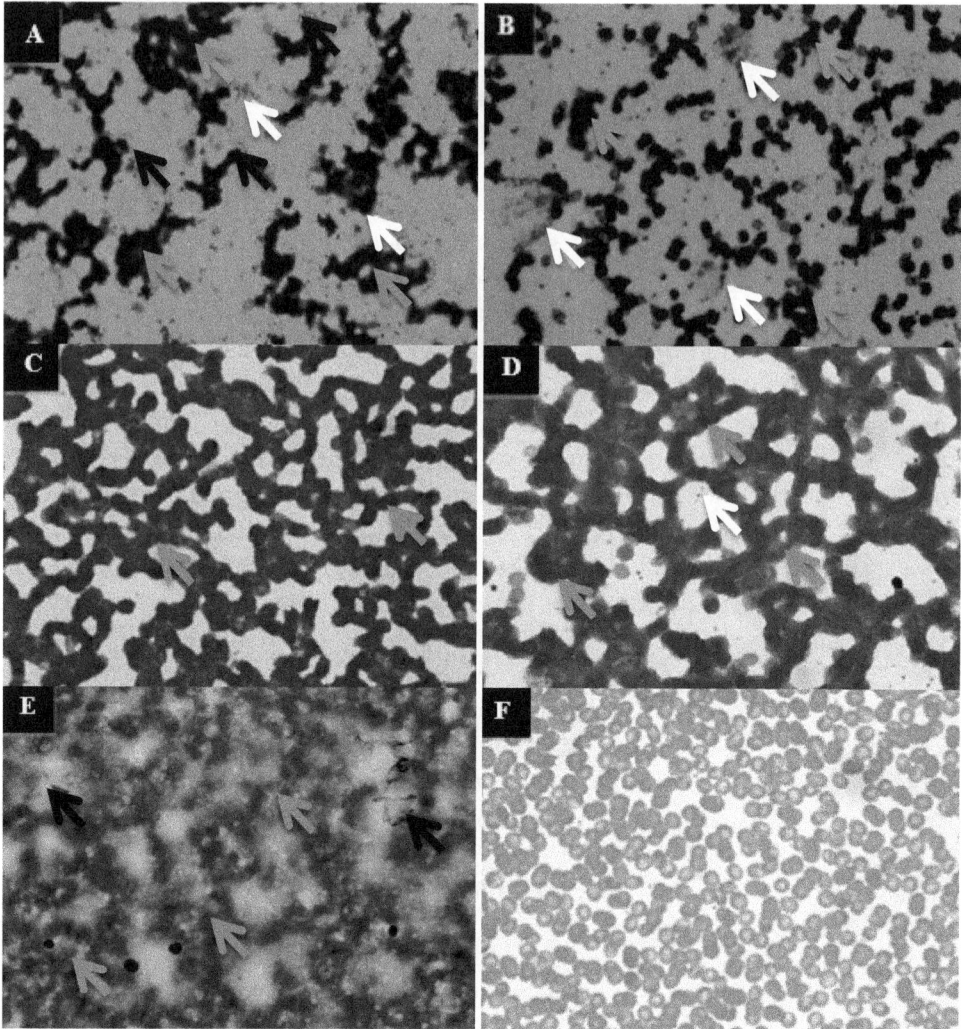

Figure 3: Erythrocyte morphology. 400× × 0.45 mm [(A) 7% NO-CMC. (B) 8% NO-CMC. (C) O-C. (D) O-C 53. (E) Lyostypt. (F) Blood alone]. The grey arrow indicates the erythrocyte aggregations, the white arrow indicates platelet aggregations and the black arrow indicates fibrin meshes.

Recent evidence suggests that chitosan-adhered blood significantly accelerates hemostasis *in vitro* by decreasing the plasma recalcification time and also by accelerating fibrin formation compared to the control groups. Platelet adherence increased and was activated on the chitosan surface membrane. Chitosan formed coagulum when it adhered to whole blood samples and was capable of aggregating without lysing the erythrocytes (Malette and Quigley, 1983; Dutkiewicz *et al.*, 1989; Rao and Sharma, 1997; Janvikul *et al.*, 2006; Periayah *et al.*, 2014). The data from several sources confirmed the finding that chito-oligomers stimulate hyaluronan synthesis, which stimulates cell adherence and proliferation towards morphogenesis, inflammation and wound healing. In another study, erythrocytes formed coagulations in the chitosan-treated lingual incisions and the morphologies were noticed to be deformation shapes (Klokkevold *et al.*, 1991; 1992). Chitosan interacted with the erythrocytes, which led to aggressive erythrocyte aggregation; at the same time, chitosan was also reported to inhibit erythrocyte lysis. The chitosan-adhered erythrocytes eventually lost their biconcave morphologies and accumulated as a clot to prevent blood flow. This study result also clearly supports the outcome hypothesizing that chitosan bio-materials are capable of promoting hemostasis by crosslinking erythrocytes together to form a lattice to ensnare the cells (Yamazaki, 2007; Periayah *et al.*, 2014). The ionic attraction between negatively charged erythrocyte membranes and positively charged groups in chitosan is one of the possible explanations for the coagulation activities of chitosan. Consequently, positively charged chitosan is more effective as a blood coagulant (Wu *et al.*, 2008).

3.2   Expression Levels of Cell Adhesion Molecules (P-Selectin) in Platelet Activation

Platelet activation usually occurs followed by platelet adhesion events. As an initial step in the platelet activation mechanism, platelets will undergo shape changes, cytoskeleton organization and organelle centralization (Ghoshal and Bhattacharyya, 2014). In the regulation of the hemostasis process, activated platelets clearly play an important role in facilitating the subsequent platelet aggregation step. However, uncontrolled platelet activation could possibly cause the blockage of vessels because of hypercoagulation.

P-selectin is also known as CD62P and is expressed in the α-granules of activated platelets and the granules of endothelial cells. It is the largest protein in the selectin family and has a total MW of 140 kDa. Endothelial cells rapidly stimulate inflammatory mediators such as P-selectin upon tissue injury. P-selectin also tends to be expressed during surgical traumas. P-selectin is rich in cysteine and contains a number of complex N-terminals, which are linked to oligosaccharides and play a significant role in platelet activation by combining with the external membrane. The expression period of the P-selectin protein is short-lived with a peak of only 10 min. The additional recruitment of P-selectin can be imparted by cytokine mediators. P-selectin mediates the interactions between the endothelium, platelets, and leukocytes by recruiting the phosphorylation of histidine residues on the cytoplasmic tail of the molecule (Crovello *et al.*, 1995). The primary ligand for P-selectin is the P-selectin glycoprotein ligand-1 (PSGL-1), which is generally found on all leukocytes. The transient interaction between P-selectin and PSGL-1 allows the leukocyte cells to move along the venular endothelium.

The P-selectin protein is also involved in the leukocyte-adhesion mechanism (Berger *et al.*, 1998). Of the multiple surface markers that can be detected upon platelet plug formation, P-selectin is one of the protein that is translocated at the outer boundary of the activated platelets. As discussed previously, chitosan is fully capable of inducing platelet adhesion by engaging in the hemostasis process. Driven by the substantial function of chitosan-derived biomaterials as an anti-hemorrhage biopolymer, the platelet activation marker P-selectin was also investigated in this study. Each chitosan biomaterial was preincubated with prepared PRP of citrated blood from healthy donors, as previously described in the methods section. A quantitative sandwich enzyme immu-noassay technique was employed. The detection range for P-selectin is 0.9 ng/mL to 60 ng/mL. The results of this study not only defined the novel role of P-selectin upon chi-tosan adhesion but also elucidated the significance of this protein towards the coagula-tion process.

Based on the assay standard operation procedure, the minimum detectable dose of human P-selectin is lesser than or equal to 0.225 ng/mL. The sensitivity of this assay, or the lower limit of detection, was defined as the lowest protein concentration that could be distinguished from 0 ng/ mL. The assay procedure that was employed also had a higher level of sensitivity and excellent specificity for detecting human P-selectin. In this test, the collected samples were stored for no longer than a week to avoid protein degradation and denaturalization, which might lead to false results.

P-selectin was continuously expressed at low levels upon adherence to different forms of chitosan. The highest mean expression level of P-selectin was induced by O-C [19.3 ± 1.61 ng/mL], followed by O-C 53 [18.5 ± 2.01 ng/mL]. Both O-C and O-C 53 showed increases of 34.7 and 31.9%, respectively, compared to blood alone. Meanwhile, the level of P-selectin increased by lyostypt with only 27.6%. Among the two tested NO-CMCs, 7% NO-CMC induced the expression level by 26.3% whereas 8% NO-CMC sup-pressed the expression level by 22.3% compared to blood alone. Comparisons have been performed between the tested groups with blood alone to elucidate any significant val-ues. Both the O-C and O-C 53 chitosan groups exhibited significant values of $p = 0.002$ and $p = 0.015$, respectively. However, the outcome result for the NO-CMC chitosan group did not show a significant value compared to blood alone (Figure 4).

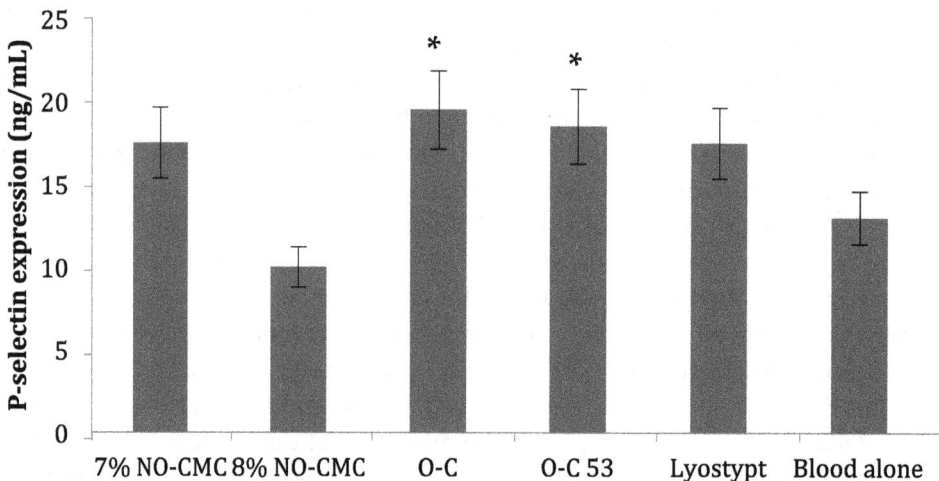

Figure 4: The mean expression of P-selectin upon the adherences of chitosan bio-materials. The error bars represent the S.E.M., and the statistically significant val-ues are clearly provided for the tested biomaterials compared to blood alone; ($n =$ 14); $p < 0.05$.

The measurement of the P-selectin protein on the platelet surface has been studied in many settings to determine platelet activation status. However, the recovery and survival of expressed P-selectin upon chitosan adherence *in vitro* is still questionable in correlation with the *in vivo* events upon tissue injury. This is because very few previous studies have been conducted to test the capability of chitosan derived hemostatic agents in inducing the P-selection protein molecule in activating platelets to assist in the hemostasis process. This study produced results corroborating the findings of many of the previous works. O-C affects thrombogenesis by changing the shape of the platelets to a pseudopodal shape, enabling aggregation (Periayah *et al.*, 2014). Therefore, this platelet activation corroborated with the platelet adhesion findings that chitosan is capable of acting on the primary step of hemostasis by improvising the platelet adherences and capillary restoration.

There are many reasons underlying the mechanism of action of P-selectin that must be studied and explored in detail to correlate this protein with platelet activity. P-selectin expression reported to stabilize the initial platelet aggregation formed by Glycoprotein IIbIIIa-Fib (GPIIbIIIa-Fib) interactions, permitting the accumulation of large aggregations. P-selectin expression upon platelet activation has the potential to determine the size and stability of platelet aggregates and to play an important role in thrombosis (Seda *et al.*, 2007). At this point, P-selectin was continuously expressed at a low level upon adherence to the various forms of chitosan, with noticeable differences in the means observed between the tested groups. Investigations of P-selectin expression in PRP might be affected by mechanical platelet activation during centrifugation (Ritchie *et al.*, 2000).

To minimize the possibility of mechanical platelet activation, three-way stopcocks were used to discard the first 1 mL of blood in the first syringe collected. Previously, it was reported that the percentage of P-selectin induced by a chitosan-heparin composite scaffold was significantly reduced compared to that induced by a chitosan scaffold alone (He *et al.*, 2010). Additionally, the levels of P-selectin were higher in platelets exposed to chitosan compared to platelets that were isolated from blood alone. The expression of the integrin GPIIbIIIa has been reported to be elevated in platelets that adhered to chitosan (Tomihata and Ikada, 1997). The expression level of P-selectin was also noted to be dependent on the type of anticoagulant used. To study this relationship, 3.2% anticoagulant tubes (K3 tubes) were used to avoid possible errors.

As formerly reported, the platelet activation stimulated by ADP or collagen was contingent on the type of anticoagulant that was used even though the minimal expression at baseline levels for all the tested samples has been described (Schneider *et al.*, 1997; Holmes *et al.*, 1999; Ritchie *et al.*, 2000). In the current study that evaluated samples without *in vitro* activation, expression was significantly higher in K3 EDTA than in sodium citrate blood. It is of note that in previous studies, K2 EDTA has been shown to upregulate the expression of P-selectin. EDTA has been well documented because it causes an upregulation of the platelet surface receptor and an increase of (McEver *et al.*, 1983), which could markedly affect the coagulation pathway. It has also been shown to cause a time dependent swelling of platelets, which leads to the denaturing and degranulation of P-selectin surface expression (McShine *et al.*, 1990; Bath 1993; Kuhne *et al.*, 1995; Golanski *et al.*, 1996; Periayah *et al.*, 2014).

3.3   Measurement of Platelet Aggregation Induced by an ADP Agonist in the Presence of Chitosan Biometerials

Platelets readily adhere on a ruptured vessel wall in response to vascular damage by stimulating a host of events that involve additional platelets to recruit for aggregation. Platelet aggregation is stimulated by the activated receptors that are conjugated with intracellular signaling, resulting in GPIIbIIIa activation. The major functions of platelets in hemostasis involve their adherences at the sites of vessel injury by activating the internal signaling pathways, which form platelet plugs to seal the injured area (Zhou & Schmaier, 2005). ADP has long been acknowledged as providing an extension of platelet activation towards vascular damage, and it is an important agonist to detect the ability of platelets to aggregate *in vivo*. Meanwhile, a platelet aggregation test can be performed utilizing whole blood and PRP by employing a few agonists that are also known as platelet activators. Scientifically, agonists are described as the chemicals or signals that adhere to the receptor by stimulating the receptor to execute a biological response.

The most common agonists used to test platelet aggregations are arachidonic acid, thrombin, epinephrine, collagen, ristocetin and ADP. These agonists can be classified into two different categories: strong and weak agonists. Thrombin, ristocetin and collagen fall under the strong agonist category because they directly induce platelet aggregation, synthesize Thromboxane A_2 (TXA$_2$) and secrete platelet granules. However, ADP and epinephrine are addressed as weak agonists because they only induce aggregation without stimulating the secretions. In this study, an ADP agonist was selected to test the level of platelet aggregation upon the adherence of the chitosan derivatives. Therefore, ADP was chosen as the agonist because platelet secretion precisely follows the aggregation that is induced by a weak agonist upon the synthesis of endogenous TXA$_2$ to be stimulated closely along platelet-to-platelet interactions throughout platelet aggregation mechanisms.

Strong agonists can potentially act as weak agonists at low concentrations, but weak agonists may not be affected even at higher concentration levels. Platelet agonist addition into blood samples can potentially activate the platelet cells by changing their shapes from a discoid pattern to spiny spheres or pseudopodal shapes, which are related to the temporary rise in the optical density of platelet aggregometry. Driven by the significant role of adherence in the platelet response during the hemostasis process, this study was conducted to evaluate platelet aggregation in the presence of ADP agonists to characterize platelet capacity with chitosan adherences. Moreover, no research has yet been conducted to test the chitosan response on platelet aggregations by adding an ADP agonist. The standard 10 μM ADP concentration was added to a chrono-log cuvette, and the results were interpreted at 5 min time intervals.

Platelet aggregation was measured using a Chronolog lumi aggre-gometer. This aggregometer measured and quantified platelet functions using electrical impedances. Generally, this is the diagnostic tool used to address the aggregation dysfunction that occurs during the hemostasis process for certain types of hemostatic abnormalities such as vWD, Bernard Soulier Syndrome and Glanzmann Thrombasthenia. The measurement of platelet aggregation also illustrates the process of dense granule release by providing better insight into the mechanisms of the platelet response.

The amplitude levels of the aggregated platelets were expressed in ohms (Ω). O-C 53 was the chitosan for which the lowest mean amplitude was reached at 1.57 ± 0.64 Ω and a difference of 11.93 Ω compared to the control level. O-C reached the second lowest level at 4.14 ± 17.71 Ω. Meanwhile, 7 and 8% NO-CMC recorded the highest amplitude release at 9.79 ± 1.30 Ω and 11.71 ± 1.18 Ω, respectively. Large differences in the mean amplitudes were noted between both the O-C and NO-CMC chitosan groups. All the tested groups of biomaterials exhibited significant differences compared to blood alone, which was only tested with the addition of ADP ($p < 0.05$; Figure 5).

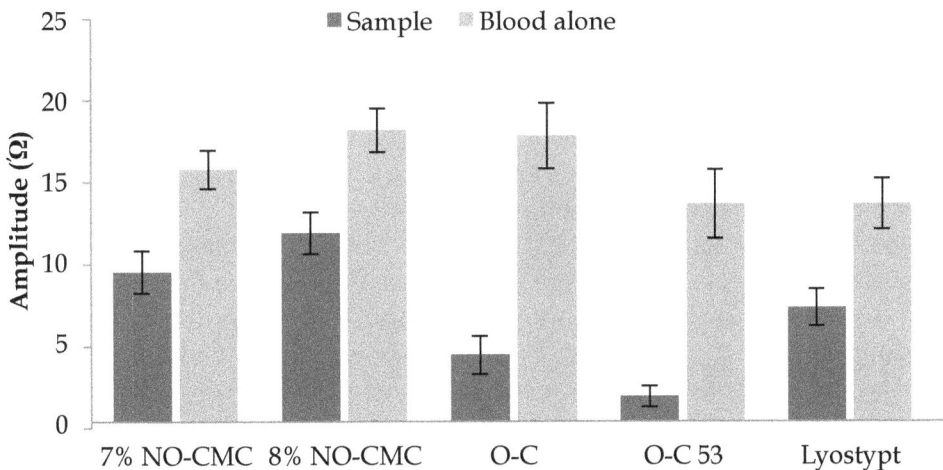

Figure 5: The mean values of chitosan-adhered platelet aggregation induced by ADP. The error bars indicate the S.E.M. ($n = 14$).

As shown in Figure 6, chitosan adhered to whole blood was stabilized first in the cuvette. The baseline of light transmission prior to the introduction of the ADP agonist is indicated by '1'. The label '2' indicates the addition of the agonist. The platelet shapes changed initially (shown by '3'), resulting in a reduction of light transmittance, followed by an initial wave of aggregation (indicated by '4'). If the stimulation of ADP is strong, a secondary wave of ADP-induced platelet aggregation occurs (indicated by '5') in which the platelet granule contents, which potentiate the primary aggregation reactions, are released. Only the results exhibited in channel number 3 are noted. This is because of the computed on-screen instructions. The slope, lag time and area under the curve were not taken into account to depict the level of platelet aggregation because they only illustrate the graph, which expresses the amplitude mode.

Although O-C 53, the powdered type of chitosan, induced a more rapid reaction among the types of chitosan studied, O-C in sponge form also registered an equivalent result. The shape change was followed by platelet aggregation and granule secretion, which led to the release of more ADP and several other substances (Mill *et al.*, 1968). ADP was used in this study because it is the best studied and most commonly used agonist. It is released from dense granules during platelet activation, and its initial binding results in the release of intracellular calcium and a change in the shapes of the platelets, leading to the primary wave of aggregation. The secondary wave reflects the release of ADP from the platelet storage granules. Low-dose ADP induces only primary aggregation, and the effect is reversible. The molecular mechanism of ADP on platelets remains unclear.

The chitosan groups O-C and O-C 53 both showed significant results, as indicated by the lowest amplitude mean levels ($p < 0.05$). This result indicates that ADP could not induce platelet aggregation because most of the platelets were attracted to chitosan, reducing the number of platelets remaining in the tested blood sample. To elaborate more on this platelet aggregation test, if the ADP stimulus was not sufficiently strong, the platelets failed to aggregate. Therefore, a comparison was performed for every sample with a negative control, which was blood alone, to ensure that the ADP agonist did not provide false positive results. To obtain optimal results, all the studies were performed within 2 hr of the blood collection. Storage time was avoided because the physiological integrity of platelets decreases with prolonged storage (Kohli *et al.*, 1998). Examples of changes in light transmission during ADP-induced platelet aggregation in the presence of O-C 53 and lyostypt are shown in Figure 6. This result showed that the O-C chitosan group performed their functions as hemostatic agents; however, these *in vitro* platelet aggregations do not precisely reflect *in vivo* platelet functions. Chitosan-adhered whole blood samples were placed in the cuvette, followed by the addition of distilled water at an equivalent ratio of 1:1. Strictly, infusion saline should not be mixed with the whole blood sample because it contains an improper osmolality, benzyl alcohol and other preservatives that could affect platelet functions. Cell counter diluents are also inappropriate to load with the whole blood for analysis because they contain EDTA, which could inhibit platelet aggregations. Although chitosan was found to form coagulum, the adherences and aggregation of the platelets did not precisely reflect blood coagulation. The effects of chitosan on the coagulation profile occur not only because of physical consequences but because of their chemical structure, particularly the amine residue (Okamoto *et al.*, 2003). This result indicates that the amine residue is important in the aggregation of platelets to form a clot (Periayah *et al.*, 2013).

In the previous morphological analysis, the membrane coverage of platelet aggregation on the surface of the chitosan scaffold was pictured clearly. At that level, the O-C chitosan group registered the biomaterials that stimulate more platelet adherences towards aggregation. ADP addition in the chitosan-adhered blood samples, which was evaluated using a turbidimetric aggregometry assessment, is one of the conformational tests used to denote and strengthen the hypothesis on platelet shape changes to form aggregation to seal an injury *in vivo*.

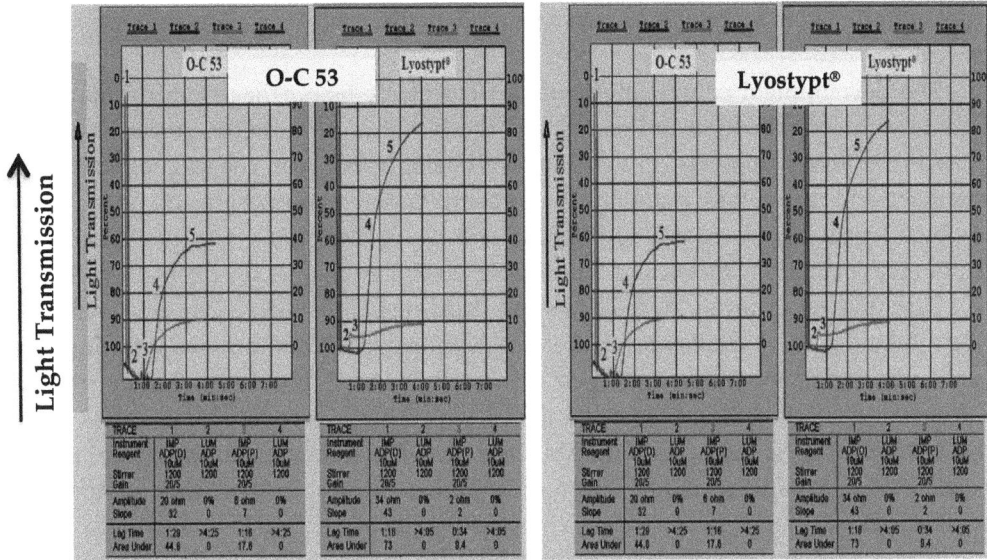

Trace	O-C 53				Lyostypt®			
	1	2	3	4	1	2	3	4
Instrument Reagent	IMP ADP(D) 10 µM	LUM ADP 10µM	IMP ADP(P) 10µM	LUM ADP 10µM	IMP ADP(D) 10µM	LUM ADP 10µM	IMP ADP(P) 10µM	LUM ADP 10µM
Stirrer Gain	1200 20/5	1200	1200 20/5	1200	1200 20/5	1200	1200 20/5	1200
Amplitude Slope	20 Ω 32	0% 0	6 Ω 7	0% 0	34 Ω 43	0% 0	2 Ω 2	0% 0
Leg Time Area Under	1:29 44.8	> 5:25 0	1:16 17.6	> 4:25 0	1:16 73	> 5:04 0	0:34 9.4	> 4:05 0

Figure 6: Examples of changes in light transmission during platelet aggregation induced by ADP in the presence of O-C 53 and lyostypt. The highlighted cells indicate the recorded amplitude (Ω) of platelet aggregation.

3.4 Effects of chitosan on coagulation ability and coagulation profiles

Hemorrhage remains the leading cause of combat death and is a major cause of death from potentially survivable injuries. Great strides have been made in controlling extremity hemorrhage with tourniquets, but not all injuries are amenable for tourniquet application. Topical hemostatic agents and dressings provide great success in controlling extremities. In many hospital settings, maintaining a good hemostatic balance in bleeding patients remains a major challenge. Successful approaches in hemostasis research may contribute to a significant reduction in hemorrhage-related fatalities. Hemostatic agents have been widely applied in surgical settings. The FDA recently issued a warning regarding a few types of hemostatic agents that had been reported to cause adverse effects such as swelling, paralysis and nerve injury because of compression (Periayah *et al.*, 2013).

The development of new methods or devices for hemorrhage control may contribute to a future reduction in hemorrhage morbidity and mortality. A successful hemostasis completely depends on the successful balance between coagulation and complementary and fibrinolytic pathways, with complex interactions between plasma proteins, blood cells, blood vessel endothelium and blood flow and viscosity (Deuel *et al.*, 1982; Berger *et al.*, 2004; Alfars and Khashjoori, 2008; Periayah *et al.*, 2013; 2014). Therefore, alternative or naturally derived wound dressings have been intensely researched to identify and resolve challenges in treating hemorrhage. Chitosan was introduced as an antihemorrhagic biomaterial because it is cationic and insoluble at a higher pH, but when reversibly sulfated, it becomes anionic, which has water-soluble properties that initiate blood coagulations (Suh and Matthew, 2000). Hence, developing novel bioadhesives and hemostatic agents has been a continued priority for reducing hemorrhage complications.

Although many studies have been conducted to clarify the hemostatic effectiveness of the application of chitosan, the hemocompatibility of chitosan derivatives still remains unexplained. In the present study, the feasibility of the chitosan biomaterials towards blood coagulation abilities and coagulation profiles were screened by employing two different methods. Whole blood and PRP were utilized to test the blood coagulation abilities. A method that mimics the Westergren method and a dynamic rheological experiment were applied to test both types of prepared blood. These classic techniques are the most common and modified methods that are applied to test the erythrocyte and PRP sedimentation rate by measuring the timed fall of the level of blood within 15 min of the time interval observed macroscopically.

This test is often referred to as a nonspecific measurement in monitoring blood diseases and assisting in a particular diagnosis. The Westergren method is not a well-understood phenomenon and can only be described in 3 different stages: aggregation, precipitation and packing. Any of the factors affecting these 3 crucial phases could possibly influence the number and shape of the blood cells and the plasma viscosity (Vennapusa *et al.*, 2011). The study of the flow of matter-like substances in solid, semi-solid and liquid conditions in which they could react favorably together with a plastic flow instead of elastic deformation upon force application is referred to as rheology (Schowalter, 1978). The rheology application between the coagulation system and the polymer surfaces of the chitosan derivatives are of a highly complex nature and largely depend on the blood compatibility of the biomaterial properties such as plasmatic enzymes, cellular elements and flowing conditions (Saito *et al.*, 1997; Kirkpatrick *et al.*, 1998; Sieminski and Gooch, 2000; Periayah *et al.*, 2014).

The blood clotting process is a host defense mechanism that helps to protect the integrity of the vascular system after tissue injury in parallel with the inflammatory and repair responses. Coagulation profile evaluations, which include APTT, PT, TT and Fib, were measured on an STA Compact Coagulation Analyzer (Diagnostica Stago, France) according to the manu-facturer's instructions. Normally, these profiles are examined in a patient with a sufficient amount of coagulation activity to ensure the blood clotting process occurs within a necessary period. Therefore, the significant of this test was to evaluate the above mentioned profile actions upon chitosan biomaterials and exhibit its effectiveness in expediting the clotting time.

3.4.1   Blood Coagulation Study

Figure 7 shows the blood coagulation ability of NO-CMC, O-C, lyostypt and blood alone. As discussed, a test that imitates the Westergren method and a dynamic rheological experiment were employed. The blood samples were allowed to settle, and blood coagulation was tested by inverting the tubes and observing erythrocyte and platelet aggregations. Upon macroscopic observation, both NO-CMC samples were able to aggregate fully within 7 min (Figure 7A, 7B). The faster aggregations were noticed because of the surface properties that influence the blood with the NO-CMC adherences. The NO-CMC surface membrane appears to be very hard and possesses a relatively greater porosity compared to the O-C chitosan group. The O-C samples fully aggregated the whole blood samples within 10 min, but for PRP, O-C was unable to fully utilize the platelets for coagulation. Within 15 min, only 75% of the PRP had been utilized, and contrary to our expectations, the powdered-type O-C 53 was able to coagulate just 50% (Figure 7D). The findings suggest that the ability of each type of chitosan to coagulate blood varies depending on its weight, thickness, hardness and tensile strength, but overall, NO-CMC and O-C were detected to promote blood coagulation but at unequal levels.

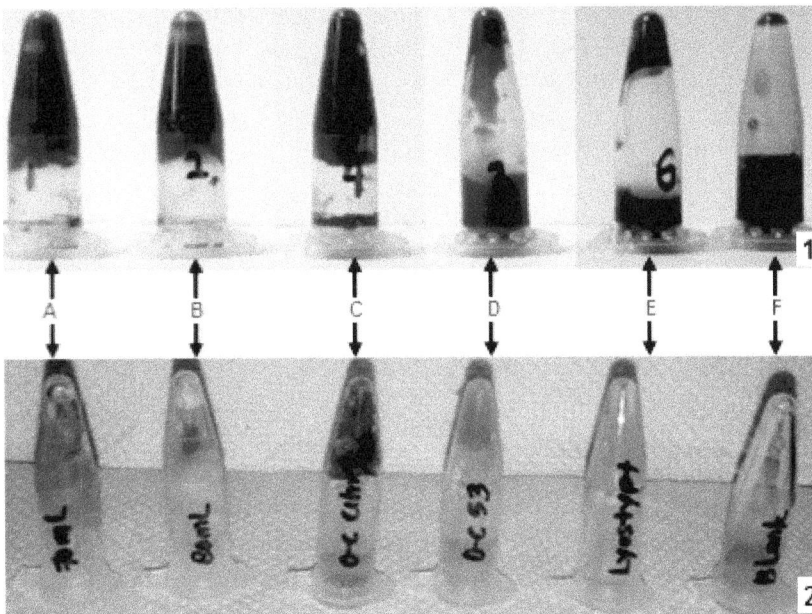

Figure 7: Blood coagulation test. (1) Whole blood coagulation. (2) PRP coagulation. [(A) 7% NO-CMC. (B) 8% NO-CMC. (C) O-C. (D) O-C 53. (E) Lyostypt. (F) Blood or PRP alone].

In the previous test that was conducted on platelet plug formation with chitosan adherences, O-C was noted to promote better platelet stimulation by engaging in the hemostasis process. The NO-CMC biomaterials were able to swell and degrade compared to the O-C group which had a positive aggregation; this was practically visible through the naked eye. Theoretically, platelet mechanical activities are believed to be concluded upon the quantification of any particular device assistances.

Chitosan is a biopolymer that is known to act on negatively charged, low-MW plasma proteins to promote aggregation (Etienne *et al.*, 2005). All the screened chitosan biomaterials in this study accelerated erythrocyte and PRP aggregation. The NO-CMCs activated the platelet and erythrocyte activities faster than O-C. O-C 53 was only partially able to aggregate erythrocytes and platelets by extending the coagulation time. The optimal biomaterial weight of 100 mg was employed, and the 7% and 8% NO-CMC were both able to aggregate 1 mL of erythrocytes or PRP within 7 min, which was consistent with a recent study by Ina Maria, 2013 in which blood in an inverted test tube became gel-like because of an increased viscosity and the presence of blood clots within 10 min of incubation with chitosan-coated films. Chitosan likely triggers hemostasis through its ionic affinity (Maria, 2013). Chitosan sponges strongly adhere to the surface membrane of muscles upon the rabbit dorsal vein wound. Throughout the implantation, the chitosan sponges were noted to promote flexibility and were resistant to wound breakage (Alfars *et al.*, 2008). This shows that chitosan did not directly injure the surface membrane of the muscle upon application and that it is possible to generate the wounded tissues. In another study, chitosan tended to expedite the bleeding time of blood drops within 2 – 2.5 min using a bandage that was dipped in chitosan solutions (Sanandam *et al.*, 2013).

Arand *et al.* reported that erythrocytes attach to one another and capture cells to build artificial clots upon chitosan adherence (Arand & Sawaya, 1986). Rao and Sharma also reported that platelets exposed to chitosan displayed a distinct adhesion to the chitosan surface within 30 to 60 sec (Rao & Sharma, 1997). This aggregation response results from the fact that chitosans are composed of glucosaminoglycan, which induces cells to adhere and form a hemostatic plug. Chitosan has also been shown to induce platelet adhesion and aggregation in a time- and concentration-dependent manner (Fischer *et al.*, 2004). Therefore, we discovered that it is possible for O-C, O-C 53 and lyostypt to coagulate to the desired level if the weight of the biomaterials is adjusted depending on their type and thickness.

3.4.2   Coagulation Profiles

The normal ranges of PT, APTT and TT in human serum are 10–21 sec, 30–45.8 sec and 11–21 sec, respectively. In this experiment, only blood alone without any biomaterial adherence expedited the coagulation times that were measured in sec. All the chitosan-adhered samples prolonged the clotting time but did not show any abnormal coagulation profile ratios. O-C 53, followed by 7% NO-CMC, was the chitosan that extended the clotting time. Followed by blood alone, lyostypt was shown to be significant by exhibiting its coagulation ability for PT within the mean period of 14.5 ± 0.67 sec; $p = 0.02$. Subsequently, O-C and 7% NO-CMC depicted a clotting period of 14.9 ± 0.45 sec; $p < 0.02$, and 15.0 ± 0.52 sec; $p = 0.01$, respectively. Although the powdered type of O-C 53 was capable of measuring the PT within the normal range, compared with all of the examined biomaterials, O-C 53 extended the PT up to 16.2 ± 0.53 sec; $p = 0.01$.

Blood alone was the best at expediting the APTT test at 39.9 ± 1.19 sec. Among the tested biomaterials, lyostypt, O-C and 7% NO-CMC were discovered to prolong the APTT profile with increases of 5.6, 6.2 and 6.3%, respectively. Meanwhile, 8% NO-CMC and O-C 53 were noted to extend the APTT outcome upon the chitosan adherences with times of 45.1 ± 1.24 sec and 45.4 ± 1.38 sec, respectively. Likewise, 8% NO-CMC and O-C 53 elucidated significant values comparable to blood alone at $p < 0.05$.

The time between the addition of the thrombin and the blood clotting was registered as the thrombin clotting time. Again, blood alone registered with a mean TT of 15.5 ± 0.49 sec, followed by O-C, lyostypt and 8% NO-CMC with recorded times of 16.7 ± 0.54 sec, 17.0 ± 0.43 sec and 18.4 ± 0.40 sec, respectively. In this test, O-C 53 and 7% NO-CMC continued to prolong the TT by 24.4% and 25.7%, respectively. All the tested biomaterials were compared to blood alone and exhibited significant values; at this level, 7% NO-CMC, 8% NO-CMC and lyostypt were demonstrated to be significant at $p < 0.05$. All the tested biomaterials were discovered to protract the coagulation profiles. A one-way ANOVA was employed to investigate the significant values between the coagulation profile groups. Significant differences were found between the tested groups for PT ($p = 0.024$), APTT ($p = 0.021$) and TT ($p < 0.05$). The asterisk (*) symbol indicates the significant values of each biomaterial compared to blood alone (Figure 8).

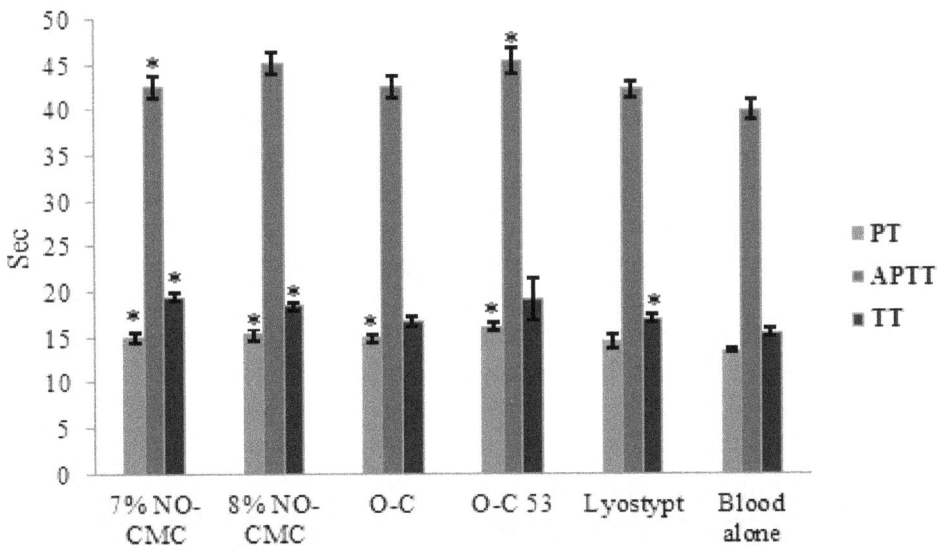

Figure 8: Coagulation profiles of PT, APTT and TT showing the means, with error bars presented as the S.E.M. The asterisk (*) symbol indicates the significant values noted compared to blood alone; ($n = 14$); $p < 0.05$.

Fib measurement was expressed in grams per deciliter (g/dL). The normal range of Fib is 14–21 g/dL. Lyostypt, O-C and O-C 53 had values of 16.6 ± 0.85 g/dL, 16.5 ± 0.84 g/dL and 16.4 ± 0.89 g/dL, respectively. Both NO-CMCs (7% NO-CMC and 8% NO-CMC) reported decreased levels of Fib by 7.1 and 9.4%, respectively, compared with blood alone. No significant differences were noted between the tested biomaterials and blood alone (Figure 9). Fib determination with thrombin clotting time originates from the method identified by Clauss. The Clauss method is a functional assay based on the time required for fibrin clot formation.

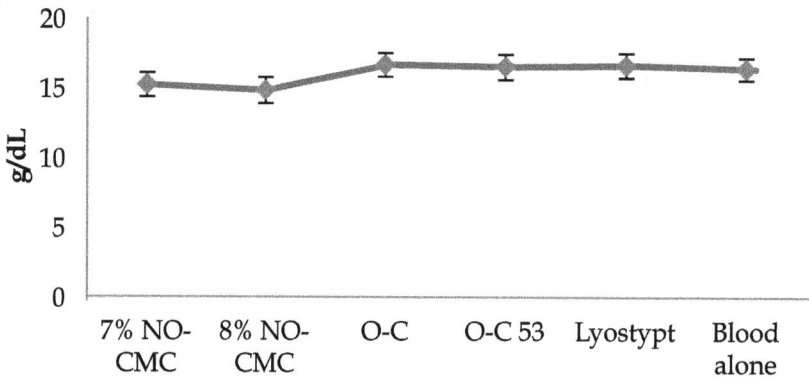

Figure 9: The mean expression of Fib of each tested biomaterial. The error bars indicate the S.E.M. (n = 14).

To complement the blood coagulation test outcomes, the coagulation profiles of PT, APTT, TT and Fib were measured. These are the parameters that are commonly measured in blood coagulation profiles to diagnose certain disorders. These tests are sensitive to both quantitative and qualitative abnormalities of any of the factors involved in the intrinsic, extrinsic and common pathways of the coagulation system. PT, APTT, TT, and Fib were measured to test the response of the intrinsic, extrinsic and fibrin formation pathways in plasma to the presence of chitosan. All the tested biomaterials promoted coagulation compared to blood alone (Figure 8 & 9). However, the findings of this study do not support the erroneous prolongation of PT and APTT levels because this test measured whole blood counts before the blood was subjected to further testing. The normal values of TT suggested that no anticoagulants were present in the blood samples. The coagulation profiles were not significantly different among the tested biomaterials, with the exception of PT. At times, PT and APTT are likely to be prolonged if the blood samples contain high levels of hematocrit (55%) or are collected in under-filled collection tubes, which is why hematocrit levels must be considered in this analysis. Therefore, the hemostasis induced by chitosan did not involve the normal blood coagulation cascade that leads to fibrin formation. In recent research, sulfated chitosan was shown to supply sufficient hemostatic effects to accelerate coagulation (Subhapradha *et al.*, 2013).

The present results are also consistent with those of other studies such as that by Romani *et al.*, who showed that sugar-modified chitosan measured by coagulation profiles did not affect coagulation pathways (Romani *et al.*, 2013), supporting the idea of chitosan-modified biomaterials functioning independently without intervening with existing coagulation mechanisms. Moreover, chitosan also sustains cell proliferation and endothelial adhesions (Khan *et al.*, 2000; Romani *et al.*, 2013), which was attributed to the physical interaction between chitosan and the cell membranes of erythrocytes. Hemostatic capacity conveyed by chitosan biomaterials enhanced only the aggregation of erythrocytes but did not accelerate the activation of the clotting time in normal coagulation pathways (Rao and Sharma, 1997). Future Fib measurement studies on chitosan could lead to a prevention of abnormal fibrinolysis in coagulopathy patients. However, the data in this study do not rule out the possible role of higher Fib levels contributing to a hypercoagulable state. The effect of chitosan biomaterials on coagulation profiles depends on their physical and chemical structure and properties, particularly the amino residues (Okamoto *et al.*, 2003). This fact is very encouraging to support our results because the biocompatible chitosans tested were found to contain *N*- and *O*- positions in their structure. In this coagulation profile study, the coagulation ability and coagulation profiles of PT, APTT, TT, and Fib upon two different groups of chitosan biomaterials were successfully demonstrated. Although the chitosan biomaterials were able to enhance the coagulation ability macroscopically, they tended to extend the examined coagulation profiles, which are the crucial screening tests for abnormal blood clotting. All the tested chitosan biomaterials recorded to coagulate within the normal clotting time range by not extending the measurement period.

4   Conclusion

Various formulations of chitosan exhibit different capabilities *in vitro* based on the chemical composition of the material. We concluded that O-C and O-C 53 were superior to other types of chitosan in achieving hemostasis. The most striking result that emerged from our present data was that O-C was superior to NO-CMC in activating platelets to form the primary hemostatic plug prior to coagulation. Novel O-C and NO-CMC were produced with varying MW, DDA and physical and chemical properties in response to different temperatures and pH levels. The platelet count noticed to decrease upon the adherences of chitosan biomaterials in a time-dependent manner and upon the addition of ADP agonist. The more the number of platelets decrease, the more the chitosan biomaterial capable to entrap platelets on the surface membrane. This suggests O-C group of chitosan have better quality for platelet adherence. O-C bound platelets formed abnormal-speculated shapes and clumped on the membrane surface layer by occupying almost 80% of the chitosan surface membrane. Irregular aggregations of erythrocytes into grape-like clusters were successfully observed for all the studied biomaterials. At the same time, O-C induced the expression level of P-selectin protein molecule indicate the prompt stimulations of platelets to activate. Both O-C and NO-CMC group of chitosan capable to coagulate within the normal clotting time range. The impact of the tested biomaterials on the coagulation depended on the physical and chemical properties of the chitosan group, particularly on the amine residues. O-Cs exert a combined effect on thrombogenesis by causing platelets to adhere, activate, aggregate and form insoluble fibrin network to strengthen platelet plug formation in normal subjects. However, NO-CMC and O-C were detected to promote blood coagulation not in equivalent level. Based on the outcome of this research, the studied novel O-C and O-C 53 stimulated hemostasis process and worked better and equal to the commercially available lyostypt. Further investigation and experimentation must be performed to determine the thickness, tensile strength, morphology and mechanical properties of the chitosan scaffolds. In the future, scaffold improvements may result in chitosan becoming the most effective naturally obtained biodegradable hemostatic adhesive yet. The relevance of these enhancements in platelet function was underscored by our current findings. Further studies are required to elucidate the precise mechanism of action of chitosan derivatives on platelets.

Acknowledgements

This project was funded by the Universiti Sains Malaysia Research Grant (RU) 1001/PPSP/813068. We thank all the donors who participated in this study.

Conflicts of Interests

The authors have declared that no competing interests exist.

References

Alfars, A.A., & Khashjoori, B.K. (2008). *Evaluation of effectiveness of chitosan hydrogel as haemostatic from dorsal nasal veins in rabbits. Basrah Journal of Veterinary Research.* 7:1.

Arand, A.G., & Sawaya, R. (1986). *Intraoperative chemical hemostasis in neurosurgery. Neurosurgery.* 18: 223–233.

Arkin, C.F., Adcock, D.M., Ernst, D.J., Marlar, R.A., Parish, G.T., Szamosi, D.I. & Warunek, D.J. (2003). *Collection, transport, and processing of blood specimens for testing plasma-based coagulation assays: approved guidelines. Wayne, PA: NCCLS.*

Bath, P.M. (1993). *The routine measurement of platelet size using sodium citrate alone as the anticoagulant. Thrombosis and Haemostasis.* 70: 687–690.

Berger, J., Reist, M., Mayer, J.M., Felt, O., & Gurny, R. (2004). *Structure and interactions in chitosan hydrogels formed by complexation or aggregation for biomedical applications. European Journal of Pharmaceutics and Biopharmaceutics.* 57: 35–52.

Berger, G., Hartwell, D.W., & Wagner D.D. (1998). P-Selectin and Platelet Clearance. Blood. 92 :11.

Bernacca, G.M., Gulbransen, M.J., Wilkinson, R., & Wheatley, D.J. (1998). In vitro blood compatibility of surface-modified polyurethanes. Biomaterials. 19:13: 1151–1165.

Cheng, T., Mathews, K.A., Abrams-Ogg, A.C.G., & Wood R.D. (2009). Relationship between assays of inflammation and coagulation: A novel interpretation of the canine activated clotting time. The Canadian Journal of Veterinary Research. 73: 2: 97–102.

Chou, T.C., Fu, E., Wu, C.J., & Yeh, J.H. (2003). Chitosan enhances platelet adhesion and aggregation. Biochemical and Biophysical Research Communications. 302: 480–483.

Crovello, C.S., Furie, B.C., & Furie, B. (1995). Histidine phosphorylation of P-selectin upon stimulation of human platelets: a novel pathway for activation-dependent signal transduction. Cell. 82: 279–286.

Deuel, T.F., Senior, R.M., Huang, J.S., & Griffin G.L. (1982). Chemotaxis of monocytes and neutrophils to platelet-derived growth factor. Journal of Clinical Investigation. 69: 1046–1049.

Dutkiewicz, J., Ludkiewzi. L., Papiewski, A.J., Kucharska, M., & Ciszewski, R. (1989). Some uses of krill chitosan as a biomaterial. Proceedings of the Fourth International Conference on Chitin and Chitosan, Trondheim, Norway. 719–730.

Etienne, O., Schneider, A., Taddei, C., Richert, L., Schaaf, P., Voegel, J.C., Egles, C. & Picart, C. (2005). Degradability of polysaccharides multilayer films in the oral environment: an in vitro and vivo study. Biomacromolecules. 6: 726–733.

Fischer, T.H., Connolly, R., Thatte, H.S., & Schwaitzberg, S.S. (2004). Comparison of structural and hemostatic properties of the poly-N-acetyl glucosamine Syvek Patch with products containing chitosan. Microscopy Research and Technique. 63: 168–174.

Garbaraviciene, J., Diehl, S., Varwig, D., Bylaite, M., Ackermann, H., Ludwig, R.J., & Boehncke, W.H. (2010) Platelet P-selectin reflects a state of cutaneous inflammation: possible application to monitor treatment efficacy in psoriasis. Experimental Dermatology. 19: 736–741.

Garcia, L.S. (2001). Diagnostic Medical Parasitology, ed. 4, ASM Press, Washington, D.C.

Gao, Y., Mansoor, A., Wood, B., Nelson, H., Higa, D., & Naugler, C. (2013) Platelet count estimation using the CellaVision DM96 system. Journal of Pathology Informatics. 4:16.

Genzen, J.R. & Milller, J.L. (2005). Presence of direct thrombin inhibitors can affect the results and interpretation of lupus anticoagulant testing. American Journal of Clinical Pathology. 124: 586–593.

Ghoshal, K., & Bhattacharyya, M. (2014). Overview of Platelet Physiology: Its Hemostatic and Nonhemostatic Role in Disease Pathogenesis. The Scientific World Journal. 781857

Golanski, J., Pietrucha, T., Baj, Z., Greger, J., & Watala, C. (1996) Molecular insights into the anticoagulant-induced spontaneous activation of platelets in whole blood - various anticoagulants are not equal. Thrombosis Research. 83: 199–216.

He, Q., Ao, Q., Gong, K., Zhang, L., Hu, M., Gong, Y., & Zhong, X. (2010). Preparation and characterization of chitosan–heparin composite matrices for blood contacting tissue engineering. Biomedical Materials. 5.

Holmes, M.B., Sobel, B.E., Howard, D.B. & Schneider, D.J. (1999) Differences between activation thresholds for platelet P-selectin and glycoprotein IIb-IIIa expression and their clinical implications. Thrombosis Research. 95: 75–82.

Janvikul, W., Uppanan, P., Thavornyutikarn, B., Krewraing, J., & Prateepasen, R. (2006). In vitro comparative hemostatic studies of chitin, chitosan, and their derivatives. Journal of Applied Polymer Science. 102: 445–451.

Jayakumar, R., Nagahama, H., Furuike, T., & Tamura, H. (2008). Synthesis of phosphorylated chitosan by novel method and its characterization. International Journal of Biological Macromolecules. 42, 335–339.

Kirkpatrick, C.J., Bittinger, F., Wagner, M., Köhler, H., van Kooten, T.G., Klein, C.L., & Otto, M. (1998). Current trends in Biocompatibility Testing. Proceedings of The Institution of Mechanical Engineers. Part H, Journal of Engineering in Medicine. 212: 2: 75–84.

Kelly, J., Ritenour, A., McLaughlin, D., Bagg, K., Apodaca, A., Mallak, C., Pearse, L., Lawnick, M., Champion, H., Wade, C., & Holcomb, JB. (2008). Injury severity and causes of death from Operation Iraqi Freedom and Operation Enduring Freedom: 2003–2004 versus 2006. Journal of Trauma. 64: S21–S26.

Khan, T., Peh, K., & Ch'ng, H. (2000). Mechanical, bioadhesive strength and biological evaluations of Chitosan films for wound dressing. Journal of Pharmacy and Pharmaceutical Science. 3: 303–311.

Khor, E., & Lim, L.Y. (2003). Implantable applications of chitin and chitosan. Biomaterials. 24: pp.2339–2349.

Kirkpatrick, J., Wagner, M., Hermans, I., Otto, M., & Bittinger, F. (1998) P.I. Haris, D. Chapman (Eds.), Endothelial–Biomaterial Interactions: A Central Role in Hemocompatibility, New Biomedical Materials, IOS Press, Amsterdam.

Klokkevold, P.R., Lew, D.S., Ellis, D.G., & Bertolami, C.N. (1991). Effect of chitosan on lingual hemostasis in rabbits. Journal of Oral and Maxillofacial Surgery. 49: 858–863.

Klokkevold, P.R., Subar, P., Fukayama, H., & Bertolami, C.N. (1992). Effect of chitosan on lingual hemostasis in rabbits with platelet dysfunction induced by epoprostenol. Journal of Oral and Maxillofacial Surgery. 50: 41–45.

Kohli, A., Khan, F., Snyder, L.M., & Pechet, L. (1998). Hemostasis Laboratory: Assays for Platelet Function and Von Willebrand Disease. Journal of Thrombosis and Thrombolysis. 6:2:159–167.

Koide, S.S. (1998). Chitin-chitosan: Properties, benefits and risks. Nutrition Research. 18: 1091–1101.

Kozen, B.G., Kircher, S.J., Henao, J., Godinez, F.S., & Johnson, A.S. (2008). *An alternative hemostatic dressing: comparison of CELOX, HemCon, and QuikClot. Academic Emergency Medicine. 215: 74–81.*

Kuhne, T., Hornstein, A., Semple, J., Chang, W., Blanchette, V., & Freedman, J. (1995) *Flow cytometric evaluation of platelet activation in blood collected into EDTA versus Diatube-H, a sodium citrate solution supplemented with theophylline, adenosine, and dipyridamole. American Journal of Hematology. 50: 40–45.*

Kuwahara, M., Sugimoto, M., Tsuji, S., Matsui, H., Mizuno, T., Miyata, S., & Yoshioka, A. (2002). *Platelet shape changes and adhesion under high shear flow. Arteriosclerosis, Thrombosis and Vascular Biology. 22: 2: 329–334.*

Lane, D. *Values of the Pearson Correlation, Statistics. Boundless, 30 Oct. 2014. Retrieved 11 Dec. 2014 from https://www.boundless.com/users/235419/textbooks/statistics/describing-bivariate-data-4/describing-bivariate-data-25/values-of-the-pearson-correlation-80-15617/.*

Laka, M., & S. Chernyavskaya, S. (2006). *Preparation of chitosan powder and investigation of its properties. Proceedings of the Estonian Academy of Sciences, Chemistry. 55: 78–84.*

Malette, W.G., & Quigley, H.J. *Method of achieving hemostasis. (1983). US Patent No. 4394373.*

Maria, I. (2013). *The synthesis of poly N-acetyl iodo glucosamine and its gelation of blood. PhD dissertation. Raleigh, NC: North Carolina State University.*

Maurer, S.E., Pfeiler, G., Maurer, N., Lindner, H., Glatter, O., & Devine, D.V. (2001). *Room temperature activates human blood platelets. Laboratory Investigation. 81: 581–592.*

McEver, R.P., Bennett, E.M., & Martin, M.N. (1983). *Identification of two structurally and functionally distinct sites on human platelet membrane glycoprotein IIb/IIIa using monoclonal antibodies. Journal of Biological Chemistry. 258: 5269–5275.*

McShine, R.L., Sibinga S. & Brozovic B. (1990). *Differences between the effects of EDTA and citrate anticoagulants on platelet count and mean platelet volume. Clinical and Laboratory Haematology. 12: 277–285.*

Merrett, K., Cornelius, R.M., Mcclung, W.G., Unsworth, I.D., & Sheardown, H. (2002). *Surface analysis methods for characterizing polymeric biomaterials. Journal of Biomaterials, Science, Polymer Edition. 13: 6: 593–621.*

Mills, D.C., Robb, I.A, Roberts, G.C. (1968). *The release of nucleotides, 5-hydroxytryptamine and enzymes from human blood platelets during aggregation. The Journal of Physiology. 195:3:715–729.*

M15-A. *National Committee for Clinical Laboratory Standards (NCCLS). (2000). Villanova, P.A.*

Muzzarelli, R.A.A., & Muzzarelli, C. (2009). *Chitin and chitosan hydrogels Handbook of Hydrocolloids (2nd ed). Cambridge UK: Woodhead Publishing. 849–888.*

Okamoto, Y., Yano, R., Miyatake, K., Tomohiro, I., Shigemasa, Y., & Minami, S. (2003). *Effects of chitin and chitosan on blood coagulation. Carbohydrate Polymers. 53: 337–342.*

Periayah, M.H., Halim, A.S., Hussein, A.R., Saad, A.Z., Rashid, A.H., & Noorsal, K. (2013). In vitro capacity of different grades of chitosan derivatives to induce platelet adhesion and aggregation. International Journal of Biological Macromolecules. 52: 244–249.

Periayah, M.H., Halim, A.S., Yaacob, N.S., Hussein, A.R., Saad, A.Z., & Rashid, A.H. (2014). Expression of P-selectin, TXA2, TGF-β1 and PDGF-AB in the Presence of Bioadhesive Chitosan Derivatives. Online International Interdisciplinary Research Journal. 4: 5–14.

Periayah, M.H., Halim, A.S., Yaacob, N.S., Hussein, A.R., Saad, A.Z., Rashid, A.H., & Ujang, Z. (2014). In Vitro comparative coagulation studies of novel biodegradable N, O-Carboxymethylchitosan (NO-CMC) and Oligo-Chitosan (O-C). International Journal of Pharmaceutical Sciences & Research. 5:11:4689–4698.

Pusateri, A.E., McCarthy, S.J., Gregory, K.W., Harris, R.A., Cardenas, L., McManus, A.T., & Goodwin, C.W. (2003). Effect of a chitosan-based hemostatic dressing on blood loss and survival in a model of severe venous hemorrhage and hepatic injury in swine. Journal of Trauma 54: 177–182.

Ritchie, J.L., Alexander, H.D., & Rea, I.M. (2000) Flow cytometry analysis of platelet P-Selectin expression in whole blood-methodological considerations. Clinical & Laboratory Hematology. 22: 359–363.

Rao, B.S., & Sharma, C.P. (1997). Use of chitosan as a biomaterial: Studies on its safety and hemostatic potential. Journal of Biomedical Materials Research: Part A. 34: 21–28

Robin, L.F., Carolyn, A.S., Stephen, R.W., Nicole, M.W., & Linda, A.D. (2012). Simple tube centrifugation for processing platelet-rich plasma in the horse. Canadian Veterinary Journal. 53: 1266–1272.

Romani A.R., Ippolito, L., Riccardi F., Pipitone, S., Morganti, M., Baroni, M.S., Borghetti, A.f., & Bettini, R. (2013). In vitro blood compatibility of novel hydrophilic chitosan films for vessel regeneration and repair. In: Pignatello R, editor. Advances in biomaterials Science and Biomedical Applications. 157–175.

Ronghua, H., Yumin, D., & Jianhong, Y. (2003). Preparation and anticoagulant activity of carboxybutyrylated hydroxyethyl chitosan sulfates. Carbohydrate Polymers. 51: 431–438.

Saito, N., Nojiri, C., Kuroda, S., & Sakai, K. (1997) Photochemical grafting of a-propylsulfate-poly(ethylene oxide) on polyurethane surfaces and enhanced antithrombogenic potential. Biomaterials. 18: 17: 1195–1197.

Salas, A. 2000. Separation of Platelets from Whole Blood. Downloaded via: http://springerlab.tch.harvard.edu/springer/uploads/Protocols/SeparationofPlateletsfromWholeBlood.pdf.

Sanandam, M., Salunkhe, A., Shejale, K., & Patil, D. (2013). Chitosan bandage for faster blood clotting and wound healing. International Journal of Advanced Biotechnology and Research. 4: 1:47–50.

Schowalter, W.R. (1978) Mechanics of Non-Newtonian Fluids Pergamon ISBN 0-08-021778-8.

Schneider, D.J., Tracy, P.B., Mann, K.G. & Sobel, B.E. (1997). *Differential effects of anticoagulants on the activation of platelets ex vivo. Circulation.* 96: 2877–2883.

Seda, R.T., Karakec, E., Menems., Gu¨mu¨¨, e., & Dereliog,˜lu. (2007). *In vitro characterization of chitosan scaffolds: influence of composition and deacetylation degree. Journal of Materials Science Materials in Medicine.* 18:1665–1674.

Sieminski, A.L., & Gooch, K.J. (2000). *Biomaterial–Microvasculature Interactions. Biomaterials.* 21: 22: 2232–2241.

Shander, A. (2007). *Financial and clinical outcomes associated with surgical bleeding complications. Surgery.* 142: 4: S20–25.

Suh, J.K.F., & Matthew, H.W.T. (2000). *Application of chitosan-based polysaccharide biomaterials in cartilage tissue engineering: a review. Biomaterials.* 21: 2589–2598.

Subhapradha, N., Suman, S., Ramasamy, P., Saravanan, R., Shanmugam, V., Srinivasan, A., & Shanmugam, A. (2013). *Anticoagulant and antioxidant activity of sulfated chitosan from the shell of donacid clam Donax scortum (Linnaeus, 1758). International Journal of Nutrition, Pharmacology, Neurological Diseases.* 3: 39–45.

Sysmex Automated Haematology Analyzer XE 5000 Instructions for use Kobe Japan, Code No. 461-2642-1, 2006–2008.

Tomihata, K., & Ikada, Y. (1997). *In vitro and in vivo degradation of films of chitin and its deacetylated derivatives. Biomaterials.* 18: 567– 575.

Turner, A.S., Parker, D., Egbert, B., Maroney, M., Armstrong, R., & Powers, N. (2002) *Evaluation of a novel hemostatic device in an ovine parenchymal organ bleeding model of normal and impaired hemostasis. Journal of Biomedical Materials Research (Applied Biomaterials).* 63: 37–47.

Vennapusa, B., La Cruz L.D., Shah H., Michalski,V., & Zhang Q.Y. (2011). *Erythrocyte Sedimentation Rate (ESR) Measured by the Streck ESR-Auto Plus Is Higher Than With the Sediplast Westergren Method A Validation Study. American Journal of Clinical Pathology.* 135:386–390.

Wagner, W., Pachence, J., Ristich, J., & Johnson, C. (1996). *Comparative in vitro analysis of topical hemostatic agents. Journal of Surgical Research.* 66: 100–108.

Wilner, G.D., Nossel, H.L., & Procupez, T.L. (1971). *Aggregation of platelets by collagen: polar active sites of insoluble human collagen. American Journal of Physiology.* 220: 1074–1079.

Wu, Y., Hu, Y., Cai, J., Ma, S., & Wang, X. (2008). *Coagulation property of hyaluronic acid–collagen/chitosan complex film. Journal of Materials Science: Materials in Medicine.* 19: 3621–3629.

Xiangmei, W., Jing, Z., Hao, C., & Qing, W. (2009). *Preparation and characterization of collagen-based composite conduit for peripheral nerve regeneration. Journal of Applied Polymer Science.* 112: 6: 3652–3662.

Yang, J., Tian, F., Wang, Z., Wang, Q., Zeng, Y.J., & Chen, S.Q. (2007) *Effect of chitosan molecular weight and deacetylation degree on hemostasis. Journal of Biomedical Materials Research Part B: Applied Biomaterials: 84B: 131–137.*

Yamazaki, M. (2007). *The chemical modification of chitosan films for improved hemostatic and bioadhesive properties. PhD dissertation. Raleigh, NC: North Carolina State University.*

Zhou, L., & Schmaier, A.H. (2005). *Platelet aggregation testing in platelet-rich plasma description of procedures with the aim to develop standards in the field. American Journal of Clinical Pathology. 123: 172–183.*

Zhou, M., Yang, J., Ye, X., Zheng, A., Li, G., Yang, P., Zhu, Y., & Cai, L. (2008). *Blood platelet's behavior on nanostructured superhydrophobic surface. Journal of Nano Research. 129–136.*

Chapter 5

Microbiota and Coronary Artery Disease

Yong Zhang[1], Heping Zhang[2]

1 Introduction

Atherosclerosis and derived CAD has been the first leading cause of death around the world (GBD 2013 Mortality and Causes of Death Collaborators, 2015). Inflammation, both systemic and peripheral, plays a key role in CAD progression (Hansson, 2005; Rein *et al.*, 2015). The rising recognition of the microbiota as a forgotten organ has been a major topic of research interest in systematic and peripheral inflammation (Purchiaroni *et al.*, 2013). Recent studies suggest that microbiota with various metabolic products are closely associated with CAD, but the detailed processes and molecular mechanisms involved remain not fully understood (Caesar *et al.*, 2010). This review will highlight the major findings and recent advances in the study of microbiota-dependent mechanism involved in the development of CAD and discuss important roles of probiotic bacteria and plant compounds in prevention and treatment of CAD.

2 CAD Featured Microbiota

In the process of atherosclerosis, it is hypothesized that CAD involved a bacterial infection and chronic inflammation of the arterial wall (Libby *et al.*, 2002). But the mechanisms of infection and related immune responses remain unexplained. In the past, the isolation of infected bacterial strain was limited to the bacterial culturing condition. By using DNA-based molecular biological techniques, bacterial and fungal DNA were

[1] Key Laboratory of Dairy Biotechnology and Engineering, Ministry of Education, Inner Mongolia Agricultural University, China
[2] Key Laboratory of Dairy Biotechnology and Engineering, Ministry of Education, Inner Mongolia Agricultural University, China

found in the atherosclerotic lesions of cardiovascular disease patients (Lehtiniemi *et al.*, 2005; Ott *et al.*, 2006; Ott *et al.*, 2007; Pessi *et al.*, 2013). A vast amount of certain microorganisms (> 50 different species), including *Chlamydia*, *Staphylococcus*, *Lactobacillus*, *Klebsiella pneumoniae*, and *Streptococcus* species, may infect the arterial wall and are associated with the development of coronary diseases (Table 1). Besides, Oral cavity derived antibiotic-resistant *Enterococcus facalis* induced infective endocarditis may have an influence on CAD development and related to high mortality (Okui *et al.*, 2015). The source of these microbes aroused great interest and were probably from oral and gut microbiota (Leishman *et al.*, 2010; Org *et al.*, 2015).

In a clinic study, CAD patients have different oral microbial flora from healthy control especially a periodontal pathogen called *Prevotella intermedia* (Nonnenmacher *et al.*, 2007). It is demonstrated that oral infective microorganisms may increase the risk of occurrence of CAD (Suzuki *et al.*, 2010). Another large-scale clinic finding revealed that periodontal microbiota was related to subclinical atherosclerosis in patients via the inflammatory C-reactive protein values (Desvarieux *et al.*, 2005). Recently, high-throughput sequencing technology may facilitate the overview of microbiota composition involved in various diseases, as well as explore the causal relationships between microbes and host. The composition of all bacteria can be more accurately evaluated by sequencing the hyper variable regions of the 16S ribosomal RNA (rRNA) bacterial gene in total DNA with next generation sequencing technologies such as Roche 454-pyrosequencing or Illumina MiSeq platform (Mardis *et al.*, 2008). The high-throughput sequencing not only explore the unculturing microbes but also providing insights into low abundances of bacteria. By using 454 pyrosequencing, the bacterial diversity in atherosclerotic plaque, oral, and gut were evaluated in patients to underscore the clinical importance of the association between microbiota dysbiosis and atherosclerotic lesions (Koren *et al.*, 2011). In fact, the various bacteria from oral and gut affects atherosclerosis far beyond our expection. More detailed, Abundances of Veillonella and Streptococcus in the atherosclerotic plaques are consistent with that in oral samples and some OTUs (operational taxonomic units) in plaques were considered gut-derived (Koren *et al.*, 2011).

Besides, blood microbiota dysbiosis was suspected to induce CAD onset in a large-scale longitudinal study by 16S rDNA sequencing. *Proteobacteria* was found to be the dominated bacteria in blood which correlated with the onset of cardiovascular complications (Amar *et al.*, 2013).

3   The Role of Microbiota in Cardiovascular Health

Previous data demonstrated that atherosclerosis-prone mice were shown no enhancement in atherscelerosis with normal diet while suppression of intestinal flora completely by antibiotic treatment (Wang *et al.*, 2011). But antibiotics treatment failed to benefit CAD in humans (Andraws *et al.*, 2005). More importantly, Stepankova *et al.*, (2010) found that germ-free ApoE-/- mice could develop atherosclerotic plaques in the aorta whereas their conventional controls had no plaques with the same diet. It is sug-

Species	Source	Role
Porphyromonas gingivalis, Aggregatibacter actinomycetemcomitans, Prevotella intermedia	Infected plaques	Periodontal disease related pathogens (Gaetti-Jardim *et al.*, 2009)
Porphyromonas gingivalis, Actinobacillus actinomycetemcomitans, Tannerella forsythensis, Eikenella corrodens, Prevotella intermedia, Staphylococcus aureus, Staphylococcus epidermidis, Streptococcus mutans, Treponema denticola, C. pneumoniae.	Atherom-atous plaques	Periodontal disease related pathogens; P.gingivalis invade human oral endo-thelial cells (Kozarov *et al.*, 2006)
Chlamydia pneumoniae	Infected plaques	Enter the bloodstream via monocytes and infect the vessel wall by leukocyte infiltration (Berger *et al.*, 2000)
Streptococcus gordonii	Oral cavities	Platelet adhesion and sub-sequent aggregation (Pe-tersen *et al.*, 2010)
Neisseria sp., Streptococcus mitis, Enterococcus sp., Lactococcus lactis sp., Haemophilus parahaemolyticus, Streptococcus pyogenes, Streptococcus salivarius, Streptococcus mitis, Prevotella sp., Lactobacillus fermentum, Lactobacillus delbrueckii	Fibroath-eroma	Enter the bloodstream dur-ing toothbrushing or by leaking through mucosal surfaces (Lehtiniemi *et al.*, 2005)
Helicobacter pylori	Atherosc-lerotic plaque	Gastric mucosal damage (Kowalski *et al.*, 2001)
Enterococcus facalis	Oral cavity	Infective endocarditis (Okui *et al.*, 2015)

Table 1: The identified CAD-associated species.

gested that gut commensal microbiota are presumed to have contributed to the prevention of atherosclerosis development. The effects of the gut microbiota on the cardiovascular health may not be limited to the presence of intestinal bacteria, but may involve
systemic immune responses driven by these bacteria. Gut microbiota appear to influence host inflammatory responses in large part by producing LPS (Lipopolysaccharides)
that enter the host circulation through impaired intestine (Org *et al.*, 2015).

Though some microbes from the oral or gut may be associated with that in atherosclerotic plaques, there no single study has directly demonstrated how the way of microbe get from their external environment to the heart to cause CAD. In my opinion,
transplantation of single risk microbe to oral or gut of germ-free ApoE-/- mice provide a
useful model to trace the way of microorganisms causing atherosclerosis. Atherosclerotic bacteria would be shown to activate inflammatory pathways, altering lipid metabolism or producing risk substances. Moreover, mice may be protected from atherosclerosis via microbiota improvement by dietary intervention.

4   TMAO and Serotonin-novel Microbiota related Factors for CAD

An earlier previous metabolomic study compared the differences in serum metabolites
between 36 severe CAD patients and 30 healthy controls. The result showed that cho-
line-containing metabolites have considerable difference in these two groups and may
used as a diagnostic biomarker (Brindle *et al.*, 2002). In recent years, trimethylamine N-
oxide (TMAO), exhibiting a strong association with CAD , has been considered as a
novel risk factor for cardiovascular disease (Tang *et al.*, 2013). Accumulating evidence
indicates that the gut microbiota can modulate the metabolism of choline to trimethylamine (TMA) and TMAO is generated from TMA via oxidization (Wang *et al.*, 2011;
Shah *et al.*, 2012). However, the core gut microbiota has not been identified to contribute
to the TMA formation.Further investigation in animals showed that dietary egg yolk
rich in phosphatidylcholine increased the TMAO levels and atherosclerosis risks, while
broad spectrum antibiotics treatment could suppress intestinal flora and prevent the
TMAO formation in mice (Tang *et al.*, 2013). It is thought that the presence of microbiota
play an obligate role in TMAO formation which is contributed to atherosclerosis risks.
Besides, a minor human study showed that daily consumption of above2 eggs that rich
in choline could increase TMAO concentrations linked with altered intestinal microbiota
composition (Miller *et al.*, 2014). It is suggest that overconsumption of eggs may increase
the risk of atherosclerosis and CAD.

Blood platelets are closely related to thrombus formation and coronary atherogenesis in the progression of CAD (Vikenes *et al.*, 1999). Yet the crosstalk between the
platelets and immune cells extends functionally far more than have been recognized
before. Platelets was also contribute to bacterial clearance in blood and thus prevention
for coronary arteries infection through the innate immune system with kupffer cells
(Wong *et al.*, 2013). Serotonin (5-hydroxytryptamine, 5-HT), secreted by platelets, are
involved in a wide range of biological functions, including vascular wall development,

thrombogenesis regulation, proliferation of smooth muscle cells and even the alleviation of comorbid depression in CAD (Pizzi *et al.*, 2011; Gershon, 2013). Over the past few years, it has become clear that gut microbiota play a role in bloodstream 5-HT levels and depression behavior by the comparison between germ-free and conventional animals (Diaz Heijtz *et al.*, 2011). Most recently, it is found that germ-free mice exhibit significantly lower levels of colonic and blood 5-HT compared to SPF controls, suggesting that gut microbiota greatly affected the 5-HT biosynthesis (Yano *et al.*, 2015). Furthermore, most of the body's 5-HT is synthesized in the gut play a key role in blood platelet activation which acted as a potential regulator in CAD prevention and development (Yano *et al.*, 2015). Another study showed that short-chain fatty acids produced by microbiota could influence the 5-HT biosynthesis by enterochromaffin cells (Reigstad *et al.*, 2015). Serotonin therefore may be one of the intestinal microbiota-dependent factors involved in the development of CAD.

5   Cholesterol: Reducing Effect of Probiotics in the Prevention of CAD

The high incidence of hypercholesterolemia imposes an enormous burden on healthcare systems and contributes to the development of atherosclerosis and related heart diseases. CAD is characterized by an imbalanced lipid metabolism and the early onset of coronary lesion is mostly independent of high circulating cholesterol level and followed by an accumulation of low-density lipoprotein (LDL) (Weber & Noels, 2011). Recent studies reveal a connection between hypercholesterolemia and microbiota (Martínez *et al.*, 2009). As a crucial player in regulating gut microbiota, some probiotics also have lipid-lowering effect (Chen *et al.*, 2013).

Mechanistically, one of main mechanisms in cholesterol -reducing is to enhance the convertion to bile acids through liver CYP7A1 activity. Another important cholesterol-reducing effect of probiotic is the direct adherence to cholesterol by bacterial cells. *Lactobacillus acidophilus* ATCC 4356, a probiotic with favorable cholesterol-reducing effect, was found to attenuate the development of atherosclerotic lesions in ApoE(-/-) mice (Chen *et al.*, 2013; Huang *et al.*, 2014). Furthermore, a comparison of intestinal microbiota between ApoE(-/-) mice with *L. acidophilus* and non- *L. acidophilus* showed significant differences in the composition of fecal lactobacillus and bifidobacterium, and these differences exhibited a correlation with inhibition of intestinal cholesterol absorption and decreased plasma cholesterol levels as well as reducing oxidative stress and inflammatory responses (Chen *et al.*, 2013). In addition, a recombinant β-glucan-producing *Lactobacillus paracasei* NFBC 338 showed a significant promotion of fecal cholesterol excretion in ApoE(-/-) mice compared to wild type strain (London *et al.*, 2014). However, obesity-preventing probiotic *L. reuteri* ATCC PTA 4659 exhibited no effects on inflammatory markers, blood cholesterol or atherosclerosis in ApoE(-/-) mice (Fåk & Bäckhed, 2012). These results indicated that, for some reason, the intestinal microbiota changes by probiotic may affect the intestinal cholesterol absorption which contribute to suppress atherosclerotic progression. However, there is controversial evidence to support the use of probiotics in patients of CAD. In one study, the findings suggest that Lactobacillus plantarum was effective for the improvement of intestinal isovaleric acid and valeric acid levels but not in blood markers in arteriosclerosis (Karlsson *et al.*, 2010). More recently, an open-label, randomized study showed *Lactobacillus casei* Shirota have limited efficacy in terms of decreasing CAD related TMAO levels in patients with metabolic syndrome (Tripolt *et al.*, 2015). Of course, more high-quality and large-scale randomized controlled trials are necessary to examine the benefits of probiotics on CAD.

6   Chloride Ion Channels in CAD Pathogensis

Although the bacterial conversion of bile acids in the human gastrointestinal tract has been well documented, the pharmacological role of various bile acids remains poorly understood (Ridlon *et al.*, 2014). It is thought that bile acid is a determinant of the gut microbiota with a high-fat diet since bile acidcould induce a rapid shift in dominating Bacteroidetes into Firmicutes (Yokota *et al.*, 2012). Because bile acids acted as a rapid response for altered gut microbiota and initiated other pathways. Bile acid sequestrants (BAS), a specific drug for eliminating bile acids in intestine, have been shown the potential role in reducing CAD progression and the risk biomarkers (Insull, 2006). In animals, the novel atherosclerotic biomarker for TMAO level is rely on liver FMOs (flavin-containing monooxygenase) expression which is mediated by the composition of bile acids (Wang *et al.*, 2011).

One of major signaling pathway for bile acids is the G protein coupled receptor TGR5. TGR5 has recently appeared to function as a target in the metabolism and inflammation of CAD (Pols *et al.*, 2011). TGR5 activation performed essential function in reducing plaque macrophage inflammation and improving atherosclerotic processes. More importantly, there exist a bile acids-TGR5-chloride ion axis where bile acids elimination and chloride ion influx were regulated by TGR5 activation (Zeng *et al.*, 2014).

Previous epidemiological survey showed that low serum chloride level had been a risk factor for cardiovascular events (De Bacquer *et al.*, 1998). Hypertension, which is more likely to develop CAD, is associated with a lower serum chloride ion concentration (McCallum, 2013). However, the underlying mechanism of low serum chloride level for risk in hypertension with CAD is unclear. It is thought that serum chloride level reflects the tissue chloride level and expression of chloride ion dependent proteins.

A series of proteins, including Cystic Fibrosis Transmembrane Conductance Regulator (CFTR), Chloride Channel-2 (ClC-2), Chloride Channel-3 (ClC-3), Chloride Channel Accessory (CLCA), Bestrophin (BEST), and Transmembrane member 16A (TMEM16A), are influenced by tissue chloride ion concentration. Previous experimental evidence has indicated that chloride ion dependent proteins may be involved in the regulation of various cellular functions, including cellular excitability, cell volume homeostasis, cell migration, proliferation, differentiation and apoptosis (Duan, 2009). *Lactobacillus casei* Zhang, a probiotic to modify the gut dominated flora, has been reported to reduce intestinal total bile acids level and enhance cardiac chloride ion concentration (Zhang *et al.*, 2014). In addition, expression of chloride ion-dependent genes ClC2, bestrophin-3 and CFTR were also upregulated with short-term probiotic intervention in heart.

Collectively, a chloride ion influx from dependence on microbiota related changes of bile acids, has been implicated in bestrophin-3 and chloride channel promotion, suggesting a potential role of probiotic in improving coronary vasomotion and preventing microvascular dysfunction during earlier CAD pathogenesis (Adkins *et al.*, 2015). Besides, cardiac CFTR over expression could modulate cell apoptosis in the basilar artery smooth muscle by regulating caspase-3 and -9 protein expression and reducing oxidative stress (Duan, 2011).

In recent years, ClC-3 has developed as a novel therapeutic target for the treatment of varous cardiac and vascular diseases (Duan, 2011). ClC-3, a chloride ion channel highly expressed in cardiac myocytes and vascular smooth muscle cells,is combined with Nox1 for some synergetic effect on reducing generation of endosomal ROS and subsequent surpress NF-κB activation by inflammatory cytokines in VSMCs. Though the relationship between ClC-3 and CAD are not clearly identified, ClC-3 may be necessary for treating inflammation and oxidative stress in CAD progression and supporting cardiac function. These considerations provided novel mechanistic insight into the beneficial effects of probiotic in the surpression of atherosclerotic process and CAD through a chloride ion influx.

Probiotics are generally defined as live microorganisms which confer health benefits when present in adequate amounts (FAO/WHO, 2001). The probiotics are considered to be strain-specific and previous research has mainly focused on the individuality of their function. In the previous studies, Lactobacillus acidophilus, Lactobacillus rhamnosus JB-1, Saccharomyces boulardii and Bifidobacterium breve C50 were found to enhance the chloride ion secretion or chloride ion related genes expression (Girard *et al.*, 2005;Heuvelin *et al.*, 2010;Raheja *et al.*, 2010;Bravo *et al.*, 2011). These experiments indicated that chloride ion-influx capacity might be a generality of probiotics. This characteristic will provide a new strategy for probiotic evaluation and consultation for probiotic related health claims.

The plant origin compounds are always considered important improvement to human cardiovascular health, and therefore identifying the mechanisms in reducing CAD is of significant interest. Plant origin compounds are always considered mostly interacted with colonic microbiota because of their relatively poor oral bioavailability and low plasma drug concentration (Cardona *et al.*, 2013). Genistein, a soy isoflavone, have shown to lower cardiovascular risk markers and in postmenopausal women with a high risk of CAD (Atteritano *et al.*, 2007). The previous report provided evidence that studies of genistein administration may exhibit increased Cl(-) secretion with activation of the CFTR chloride channel and thereby contribute to significant increases in basal I(sc) associated with intestinal epithelia function (Al-Nakkash *et al.*, 2006; Tuo *et al.*, 2009; Al-Nakkash *et al.*, 2011). In addition, genistein have a direct influence on gut dominant communities and are amenable to further bacterial metabolism to yield equol and 5-hydroxy-equol via altered microbiota in postmenopausal women (Clavel *et al.*, 2005; Matthies *et al.*, 2012). These researches suggest that genistein might have a potential beneficial role in reducing CAD by regulation of microbiota and related intestinal chloride ion proteins. Curcumin, another plant compound from curry powder, was also shown to ameliorate the development of cardiovascular diseases and stimulate CFTR Cl(-) channels directly (Berger *et al.,* 2005;Wongcharoen *et al.,* 2009; Bernard *et al.,* 2009).

Dihydromyricetin, an abundant ingredient in rattan tea, was reported to possess anti-inflammatory, antimicrobial activity, and can protect vein endothelial cells from oxidative stress damage, an effect that is potential to reduce the risk of CAD involving the mitochondrial pathways (Kou & Chen, 2012; Hou *et al.,* 2015). More importantly, dihydromyricetin affected the expression of chloride ion-dependent GABA receptors protein in brain tissue to exert beneficial effect on alcohol intoxication and Alzheimer's disease (Shen *et al.,* 2012; Liang *et al.,* 2014). These researches suggest that plant origin compounds may influence the whole body chloride ion movement not only be limited to intestine.

7　Conclusion

In this chapter, we summarized the CAD featured microbes, the oral or gut microbiota in cardiovascular health and described the potential role of bacterial metabolites such as TMAO and serotonin in the CAD pathogenicity. Though the underlying role and inter-action of numerous CAD related microbes in CAD has been not fully understood, the causal relationship of bacterial metabolite TMAO and cardiovascular disease become more clearly. In addition, serotonin may act as a potential regulator in CAD development. Moreover, importance of probiotic as a cholesterol regulator in the control of CAD development and related mechanism was recalled. Cholesterol-reducing effect of probiotics is linked to CYP7A1 activity and bacterial adherence to cholesterol.

The identity and physiological roles of chloride ion channels and proteins has lagged behind that of many other drug targets (Verkman & Galietta, 2009). Bile acids and its receptor TGR5 affected by gut microbiota could influence the secretion of chloride ion and expression of chloride ion channels. The deficit of chloride ion channels function may be responsible for the altered microbiota and metabolic disturbance in response to cholesterol-rich diet, implicating a novel and important role of chloride ion channels in the development of CAD. Recently, targeted chloride ion related proteins regulated by probiotics or plant compounds seem have relevance to the suppression of CAD. In future, multiple omics view may provide a more complete understanding of the chloride ion-dependent gene function for CAD prevention in the context of microbiota changes.

Refernces

Adkins, G.B., Curtis, M.J. (2015). *Potential role of cardiac chloride channels and transporters as novel therapeutic targets. Pharmacol Ther, 145:67–75.*

Al-Nakkash, L., Clarke, L.L., Rottinghaus, G.E., Chen, Y.J., Cooper, K., Rubin, L.J. (2006).Dietary genistein stimulates anion secretion across female murine intestine. J Nutr, 136(11):2785–2790.

Al-Nakkash, L., Batia, L., Bhakta, M., Peterson, A., Hale, N., Skinner, R., Sears, S., Jensen, J. (2011). Stimulation of murine intestinal secretion by daily genistein injections: gender-dependent differences. Cell Physiol Biochem, 28(2):239–250.

Amar, J., Lange, C., Payros, G., Garret, C., Chabo, C., Lantieri, O., Courtney, M., Marre, M., Charles, M.A., Balkau, B., Burcelin, R., D.E.S.I.R. Study Group. (2013). Blood microbiota dysbiosis is associated with the onset of cardiovascular events in a large general population: the D.E.S.I.R. study. PLoS One, 8(1):e54461.

Andraws, R., Berger, J.S., Brown, D.L. (2005). Effects of antibiotic therapy on outcomes of patients with coronary artery disease: a meta-analysis of randomized controlled trials. JAMA, 293:2641–2647.

Atteritano, M., Marini, H., Minutoli, L., Polito, F., Bitto, A., Altavilla, D., Mazzaferro, S., D'Anna, R., Cannata, M.L., Gaudio, A., Frisina, A., Frisina, N., Corrado, F., Cancellieri, F., Lubrano, C., Bonaiuto, M., Adamo, E.B., Squadrito, F. (2007). Effects of the phytoestrogen genistein on some predictors of cardiovascular risk in osteopenic, postmenopausal women: a two-year randomized, double-blind, placebo-controlled study. J Clin Endocrinol Metab, 92(8):3068–3075.

Berger, M., Schröder, B., Daeschlein, G., Schneider, W., Busjahn, A., Buchwalow, I., Luft, F,C,, Haller, H. (2000). Chlamydia pneumoniae DNA in non-coronary atherosclerotic plaques and circulating leukocytes. J Lab Clin Med, 136(3):194–200.

Berger, A.L., Randak, C.O., Ostedgaard, L.S., Karp, P.H., Vermeer, D.W., Welsh, M.J. (2005). Curcumin stimulates cystic fibrosis transmembrane conductance regulator Cl- channel activity. J Biol Chem, 280(7):5221–5226.

Bernard, K., Wang, W., Narlawar, R., Schmidt, B., Kirk, K.L. (2009). Curcumin cross-links cystic fibrosis transmembrane conductance regulator (CFTR) polypeptides and potentiates CFTR channel activity by distinct mechanisms. J Biol Chem, 284(45):30754–30765.

Bravo, J.A., Forsythe, P., Chew, M.V., Escaravage, E., Savignac, H.M., Dinan, T.G., Bienenstock, J., Cryan, J.F. (2011). Ingestion of Lactobacillus strain regulates emotional behavior and central GABA receptor expression in a mouse via the vagus nerve. ProcNatlAcadSci U S A, 108:16050–16055;

Brindle, J.T., Antti, H., Holmes, E., Tranter, G., Nicholson, J.K., Bethell, H.W., Clarke, S., Schofield, P.M., McKilligin, E., Mosedale, D.E., Grainger, D.J. (2002). Rapid and noninvasive diagnosis of the presence and severity of coronary heart disease using 1H-NMR-based metabonomics.Nat Med, 8:1439–1444.

Caesar, R., Fåk, F., Bäckhed, F. (2010).Effects of gut microbiota on obesity and atherosclerosis via modulation of inflammation and lipid metabolism. J Intern Med, 268(4):320–328.

Cardona, F., Andrés-Lacueva, C., Tulipani, S., Tinahones, F.J., Queipo-Ortuño, M.I. (2013). Benefits of polyphenols on gut microbiota and implications in human health. J Nutr Biochem, 24(8):1415–22.

Chen, L., Liu, W., Li, Y., Luo, S., Liu, Q., Zhong, Y., Jian, Z., Bao, M. (2013). Lactobacillus acidophilus ATCC 4356 attenuates the atherosclerotic progression through modulation of oxidative stress and inflammatory process. Int Immunopharmacol, 17(1):108–115.

Clavel, T., Fallani, M., Lepage, P., Levenez, F., Mathey, J., Rochet, V., Sérézat, M., Sutren, M., Henderson, G., Bennetau-Pelissero, C., Tondu, F., Blaut, M., Doré, J., Coxam, V. (2005). Isoflavones and functional foods alter the dominant intestinal microbiota in postmenopausal women. J Nutr, 135(12):2786–2792.

De Bacquer, D., De Backer, G., De Buyzere, M., Kornitzer, M. (1998). Is low serum chloride level a risk factor for cardiovascular mortality? J Cardiovasc Risk, 5(3):177–184.

Desvarieux, M., Demmer, R.T., Rundek, T., Boden-Albala, B., Jacobs, D.R., Sacco, R.L., Papapanou, P.N. (2005). Periodontal microbiota and carotid intima-media thickness: the Oral Infections and Vascular Disease Epidemiology Study (INVEST). Circulation, 111(5):576–582.

Diaz Heijtz, R., Wang, S., Anuar, F., Qian, Y., Björkholm, B., Samuelsson, A., Hibberd, M.L., Forssberg, H., Pettersson, S. (2011). Normal gut microbiota modulates brain development and behavior.Proc Natl Acad Sci U S A, 108(7):3047–3052.

Duan,D. (2009).Phenomics of cardiac chloride channels: the systematic study of chloride channel function in the heart. J Physiol, 58:2163–2177.

Duan, D.D. (2011). The ClC-3 chloride channels in cardiovascular disease. Acta Pharmacol Sin, 32(6):675–684.

Gaetti-Jardim, E., Marcelino, S.L., Feitosa, A.C., Romito, G.A., Avila-Campos, M.J. (2009).Quantitative detection of periodontopathic bacteria in atherosclerotic plaques from coronary arteries. J Med Microbiol, 58:1568–1575.

GBD 2013 Mortality and Causes of Death Collaborators.(2015). Global, regional, and national age-sex specific all-cause and cause-specific mortality for 240 causes of death, 1990–2013: a systematic analysis for the Global Burden of Disease Study 2013. Lancet, 385(9963):117–171.

Gershon, M.D. (2013).5-Hydroxytryptamine (serotonin) in the gastrointestinal tract.Curr Opin Endocrinol Diabetes Obes, 20(1):14–21.

Fåk, F., Bäckhed, F. (2012). Lactobacillus reuteri prevents diet-induced obesity, but not atherosclerosis, in a strain dependent fashion in Apoe-/- mice. PLoS One, 7(10):e46837.

FAO/WHO. (2001). Health and nutritional properties of probioticsin food including powder milk with livelactic acid bacteria. Cordoba, Argentina. ftp://ftp.fao.org/es/esn/food/probio_report_en.pdf

Girard, P., Pansart, Y., Coppe, M.C., Gillardin, J.M. (2005). *Saccharomyces boulardii inhibits water and electrolytes changes induced by castor oil in the rat colon*. Dig Dis Sci, 50:2183–2190.

Hansson, G.K. (2005). *Inflammation, atherosclerosis, and coronary artery disease*. N Engl J Med, 352(16):1685–1695.

Heuvelin, E., Lebreton, C., Bichara, M., Cerf-Bensussan, N., Heyman, M. (2010). *A Bifidobacterium probiotic strain and its soluble factors alleviate chloride secretion by human intestinal epithelial cells*. J Nutr, 140:7–11.

Hou, X., Tong, Q., Wang, W., Xiong, W., Shi, C., Fang, J. (2015). *Dihydromyricetin protects endothelial cells from hydrogen peroxide-induced oxidative stress damage by regulating mitochondrial pathways*. Life Sci, 130(1):38–46.

Huang, Y., Wang, J., Quan, G., Wang, X., Yang, L., Zhong, L. (2014). *Lactobacillus acidophilus ATCC 4356 prevents atherosclerosis via inhibition of intestinal cholesterol absorption in apolipoprotein E-knockout mice*. Appl Environ Microbiol, 80(24):7496–504.

Insull, W. (2006). *Clinical utility of bile acid sequestrants in the treatment of dyslipidemia: a scientific review*. South Med J, 99(3):257–273.

Karlsson, C., Ahrné, S., Molin, G., Berggren, A., Palmquist, I., Fredrikson, G.N., Jeppsson, B. (2010). *Probiotic therapy to men with incipient arteriosclerosis initiates increased bacterial diversity in colon: a randomized controlled trial*. Atherosclerosis, 208(1):228–233.

Koren, O., Spor, A., Felin, J., Fåk, F., Stombaugh, J., Tremaroli, V., Behre, C.J., Knight, R., Fagerberg, B., Ley, R.E., Bäckhed, F. (2011). *Human oral, gut, and plaque microbiota in patients with atherosclerosis*. Proc Natl Acad Sci U S A, 108 Suppl 1:4592–4598.

Kou, X., Chen, N. (2012). *Pharmacological potential of ampelopsin in Rattan tea*. Food Sci Human Wellness, 1(1):14–18.

Kowalski, M. Helicobacter pylori (H. pylori) *infection in coronary artery disease*: (2001). *influence of H. pylori eradication on coronary artery lumen after percutaneous transluminal coronary angioplasty. The detection of H. pylori specific DNA in human coronary atherosclerotic plaque*. J Physiol Pharmacol, 52(1 Suppl 1):3–31.

Kozarov, E., Sweier, D., Shelburne, C., Progulske-Fox, A., Lopatin, D. (2006). *Detection of bacterial DNA in atheromatous plaques by quantitative PCR*. Microbes Infect, 8(3):687–693.

Liang, J., López-Valdés, H.E., Martínez-Coria, H., Lindemeyer, A.K., Shen, Y., Shao, X.M., Olsen, R.W. (2014). *Dihydromyricetin ameliorates behavioral deficits and reverses neuropathology of transgenic mouse models of Alzheimer's disease*. Neurochem Res, 39(6):1171–1181.

Lehtiniemi, J., Karhunen, P.J., Goebeler, S., Nikkari, S., Nikkari, S.T. (2005). *Identification of different bacterial DNAs in human coronary arteries*. Eur J Clin Invest, 35(1):13–16.

Leishman, S.J., Do, H.L., Ford, P.J. (2010). *Cardiovascular disease and the role of oral bacteria*. J Oral Microbiol, 2

Libby, P., Ridker, P.M., Maseri, A. (2002). Inflammation and atherosclerosis.Circulation, 105(9):1135–1143.

London, L.E., Kumar, A.H., Wall, R., Casey, P.G., O'Sullivan, O., Shanahan, F., Hill, C., Cotter, P.D., Fitzgerald, G.F., Ross, R.P., Caplice, N.M., Stanton, C. (2014). Exopolysaccharide-producing probiotic Lactobacilli reduce serum cholesterol and modify enteric microbiota in ApoE-deficient mice. J Nutr, 144(12):1956–1962.

Matthies, A., Loh, G., Blaut, M., Braune, A. (2012).Daidzein and genistein are converted to equol and 5-hydroxy-equol by human intestinal Slackia isoflavoniconvertens in gnotobiotic rats. J Nutr,142(1):40–46.

Mardis, E.R. (2008). Next-generation DNA sequencing methods. Annu Rev Genomics Hum Genet, 9:387–402.

Martínez, I., Wallace, G., Zhang, C., Legge, R., Benson, A.K., Carr, T.P., Moriyama, E.N., Walter, J. (2009). Diet-induced metabolic improvements in a hamster model of hypercholesterolemia are strongly linked to alterations of the gut microbiota.Appl Environ Microbiol, 75(12):4175–4184.

McCallum, L., Jeemon, P., Hastie, C.E., Patel, R.K., Williamson, C., Redzuan, A.M., Dawson, J., Sloan, W., Muir, S., Morrison, D., McInnes, G.T., Freel, E.M., Walters, M., Dominiczak, A.F., Sattar, N., Padmanabhan, S. (2013). Serum chloride is an independent predictor of mortality in hypertensive patients. Hypertension, 62(5):836–843.

Miller, C.A., Corbin, K.D., da Costa, K.A., Zhang, S., Zhao, X., Galanko, J.A., Blevins, T., Bennett, B.J., O'Connor, A., Zeisel, S.H. (2014). Effect of egg ingestion on trimethylamine-N-oxide production in humans: a randomized, controlled, dose-response study. Am J ClinNutr, 100(3):778–786.

Nonnenmacher, C., Stelzel, M., Susin, C., Sattler, A.M., Schaefer, J.R., Maisch, B., Mutters, R., Flores-de-Jacoby, L. (2007). Periodontal microbiota in patients with coronary artery disease measured by real-time polymerase chain reaction: a case-control study. J Periodontol, 78(9):1724–1730.

Okui, A., Soga, Y., Kokeguchi, S., Nose, M., Yamanaka, R., Kusano, N., Morita, M. (2015). Detection of Identical Isolates of Enterococcus faecalis from the Blood and Oral Mucosa in a Patient with Infective Endocarditis. Intern Med, 54:1809–1814.

Org, E., Mehrabian, M., Lusis, A.J. (2015). Unraveling the environmental and genetic interactions in atherosclerosis: Central role of the gut microbiota. Atherosclerosis, 241(2):387–399.

Ott, S.J., El Mokhtari, N.E., Musfeldt, M., Hellmig, S., Freitag, S., Rehman, A., Kühbacher, T., Nikolaus, S., Namsolleck, P., Blaut, M., Hampe, J., Sahly, H., Reinecke, A., Haake, N., Günther, R., Krüger, D., Lins, M., Herrmann, G., Fölsch, U.R., Simon, R., Schreiber, S. (2006). Detection of diverse bacterial signatures in atherosclerotic lesions of patients with coronary heart disease. Circulation, 113(7):929–937.

Ott, S.J., El Mokhtari, N.E., Rehman, A., Rosenstiel, P., Hellmig, S., Kühbacher, T., Lins, M., Simon, R., Schreiber, S. (2007). Fungal rDNA signatures in coronary atherosclerotic plaques. Environ Microbiol, 9(12):3035–3045.

Pessi, T., Karhunen, V., Karjalainen, P.P., Ylitalo, A., Airaksinen, J.K., Niemi, M., Pietila, M., Lounatmaa, K., Haapaniemi, T., Lehtimäki, T., Laaksonen, R., Karhunen, P.J., Mikkelsson, J. (2013). Bacterial signatures in thrombus aspirates of patients with myocardial infarction.Circulation, 127(11):1219–1228.

Petersen, H.J., Keane, C., Jenkinson, H.F., Vickerman, M.M., Jesionowski, A., Waterhouse, J.C., Cox, D., Kerrigan, S.W. (2010). Human platelets recognize a novel surface protein, PadA, on Streptococcus gordonii through a unique interaction involving fibrinogen receptor GPIIbIIIa. Infect Immun, 78(1):413–422.

Pizzi, C., Rutjes, A.W., Costa, G.M., Fontana, F., Mezzetti, A., Manzoli, L. (2011). Meta-analysis of selective serotonin reuptake inhibitors in patients with depression and coronary heart disease. Am J Cardiol, 107(7):972–979.

Pols, T.W., Nomura, M., Harach, T., Lo Sasso, G., Oosterveer, M.H., Thomas, C., Rizzo, G., Gioiello, A., Adorini, L., Pellicciari, R., Auwerx, J., Schoonjans, K. (2011). TGR5 activation inhibits atherosclerosis by reducing macrophage inflammation and lipid loading. Cell Metab, 14(6):747–757.

Purchiaroni, F., Tortora, A., Gabrielli, M., Bertucci, F., Gigante, G., Ianiro, G., Ojetti, V., Scarpellini, E., Gasbarrini, A. (2013). The role of intestinal microbiota and the immune system. Eur Rev Med Pharmacol Sci, 17(3):323–333.

Raheja, G., Singh, V., Ma, K., Boumendjel, R., Borthakur, A., Gill, R.K., Saksena, S., Alrefai, W.A., Ramaswamy, K., Dudeja, P.K. (2010). Lactobacillus acidophilus stimulates the expression of SLC26A3 via a transcriptional mechanism. Am J Physiol Gastrointest Liver Physiol, 298: 395–401.

Reigstad, C.S.,Salmonson, C.E., Rainey, J.F., Szurszewski, J.H., Linden, D.R., Sonnenburg, J.L., Farrugia, G., Kashyap, P.C. (2015). Gut microbes promote colonic serotonin production through an effect of short-chain fatty acids on enterochromaffin cells. FASEB J, 29(4):1395–403.

Rein, P., Saely, C.H., Silbernagel, G., Vonbank, A., Mathies, R., Drexel, H., Baumgartner, I. (2015). Systemic inflammation is higher in peripheral artery disease than in stable coronary artery disease. Atherosclerosis, 239(2):299–303.

Ridlon, J.M., Kang, D.J., Hylemon, P.B., Bajaj, J.S. (2014). Bile acids and the gut microbiome. Curr Opin Gastroenterol, 30(3):332–338.

Shah, S.H., Kraus, W.E., Newgard, C.B. (2012). Metabolomic profiling for the identification of novel biomarkers and mechanisms related to common cardiovascular diseases: form and function. Circulation, 126(9):1110–11120.

Shen, Y., Lindemeyer, A.K., Gonzalez, C., Shao, X.M., Spigelman, I., Olsen, R.W., Liang, J. (2012). Dihydromyricetin as a novel anti-alcohol intoxication medication. J Neurosci, 32(1):390–401.

Stepankova, R., Tonar, Z., Bartova, J., Nedorost, L., Rossman, P., Poledne, R., Schwarzer, M., Tlaskalova-Hogenova, H. (2010). Absence of microbiota (germ-free conditions) accelerates the atherosclerosis in ApoE-deficient mice fed standard low cholesterol diet. J Atheroscler Thromb, 17(8):796–804.

Suzuki, J., Aoyama, N., Ogawa, M., Hirata, Y., Izumi, Y., Nagai, R., Isobe, M. (2010). Periodontitis and cardiovascular diseases. Expert Opin Ther Targets, 14:1023–1027.

Tang, W.H., Wang, Z., Levison, B.S., Koeth, R.A., Britt, E.B., Fu, X., Wu, Y., Hazen, S.L. (2013).Intestinal microbial metabolism of phosphatidylcholine and cardiovascular risk. N Engl J Med, 368(17):1575–1584.

Tripolt, N.J., Leber, B., Triebl, A., Köfeler, H., Stadlbauer, V., Sourij, H. (2015). Effect of Lactobacillus casei Shirota supplementation on trimethylamine-N-oxide levels in patients with metabolic syndrome: An open-label, randomized study. Atherosclerosis, 242(1):141–144.

Tuo, B., Wen, G., Seidler, U. (2009). Differential activation of the HCO(3)(-) conductance through the cystic fibrosis transmembrane conductance regulator anion channel by genistein and forskolin in murine duodenum. Br J Pharmacol, 158(5):1313–1321.

Verkman, A.S., Galietta, L.J. (2009). Chloride channels as drug targets. Nat Rev Drug Discov, 8(2):153–171.

Vikenes, K., Farstad, M., Nordrehaug, J.E. (1999). Serotonin is associated with coronary artery disease and cardiac events.Circulation, 100(5):483–489.

Wang, Z., Klipfell, E., Bennett, B.J., Koeth, R., Levison, B.S., Dugar, B., Feldstein, A.E., Britt, E.B., Fu, X., Chung, Y.M., Wu, Y., Schauer, P,, Smith, J.D., Allayee, H., Tang, W.H., DiDonato, J.A., Lusis, A.J., Hazen, S.L. (2011). Gut flora metabolism of phosphatidylcholine promotes cardiovascular disease. Nature, 472(7341):57–63.

Weber, C., Noels, H. (2011). Atherosclerosis: current pathogenesis and therapeutic options.Nat Med, 17(11):1410–1422.

Wong, C.H., Jenne, C.N., Petri, B., Chrobok, N.L., Kubes, P. (2013). Nucleation of platelets with blood-borne pathogens on Kupffer cells precedes other innate immunity and contributes to bacterial clearance. Nat Immunol, 14(8):785–792.

Wongcharoen, W., Phrommintikul, A. (2009).The protective role of curcumin in cardiovascular diseases. Int J Cardiol, 133(2):145–151.

Yano, J.M., Yu, K., Donaldson, G.P., Shastri, G.G., Ann, P., Ma, L., Nagler, C.R., Ismagilov, R.F., Mazmanian, S.K., Hsiao, E.Y. (2015). Indigenous bacteria from the gut microbiota regulate host serotonin biosynthesis. Cell, 161(2):264–276.

Yokota, A., Fukiya, S., Islam, K.B., Ooka, T., Ogura, Y., Hayashi, T., Hagio, M., Ishizuka, S. (2012). Is bile acid a determinant of the gut microbiota on a high-fat diet? Gut Microbes, 3(5):455–459.

Zeng, J.W., Zeng, X.L., Li, F.Y., Ma, M.M., Yuan, F., Liu, J., Lv, X.F., Wang, G.L., Guan, Y.Y. (2014). Cystic Fibrosis Transmembrane Conductance Regulator (CFTR) prevents apoptosis *induced by hydrogen peroxide in basilar artery smooth muscle cells. Apoptosis, 19(9):1317–1329.*

Zhang, Y., Guo, X., Guo, J., He, Q., Li, H., Song, Y., Zhang, H. (2014). Lactobacillus casei reduces susceptibility to type 2 diabetes via microbiota-mediated body chloride ion influx. Sci Rep, 4:5654.

Chapter 6

Resting Heart Rate Significance in the Pathogenesis, Management and Prevention of Coronary Artery Disease

Antoine Kossaify[1]

1 Background

1.1 Introduction

Coronary artery disease (CAD) represents a major cause of morbidity and mortality worldwide and its high prevalence is a real public health burden nowadays. The resting heart rate (RHR) represents the heart rate (HR) value at rest and it is an important clinical parameter useful as valuable marker in the management of many cardiovascular conditions such as heart failure, CAD and hypertension. The impact of increased RHR (iRHR) on the pathogenesis of cardiovascular diseases has been referred to almost 20 years ago, however, RHR remains poorly implemented nowadays for prevention and management of cardiovascular diseases (Tardif, 2009).

For instance, iRHR is a marker of adverse outcome in patients with heart failure, also it is a marker of increased sympathetic activity in essential hypertension and is associated with adverse events (Kannel *et al.*, 1987). Nevertheless, little attention is generally given to RHR in patients with heart failure or with hypertension, and we estimate that what is classically considered "normal" HR needs probably to be redefined. In view of this, we consider that RHR is a relatively "neglected" parameter in the armamentarium used to decrease the burden of cardiovascular diseases nowadays.

CAD is the number one cause of cardiac morbidity and mortality worldwide, despite all the medical and technical advancements brought in terms of prevention and

[1] Cardiology Department, University Hospital, Holy Spirit University of Kaslik (USEK), Lebanon

treatment; in view of this, management of CAD must be conceived as a whole process starting from primary prevention and early diagnosis, through drug and technical therapy until secondary prevention; through all these stages, HR control (HRC) is of utmost importance for a better prevention and management of CAD. In this chapter, we meant by iRHR a HR ≥70 bpm, and HRC aims basically to keep RHR below 70 bpm.

1.2   Heart Rate and Longevity

HR value has been associated with longevity in many animal and human studies and the "heartbeat" hypothesis postulates that every living creature has a limited number of heart beats predetermined by basic energetics where HR is a marker of the metabolic rate (stessman *et al.*, 2013; Speakman *et al.*, 2002). An inverse semi-logarithmic relation exists between HR and life expectancy, and the basal energy consumption/body atom directly affects HR in all animals, supporting the theory of "heartbeat" regarding HR and longevity (Levine, 1997). The "heartbeat" hypothesis is based on two observations: first, the so-called "mouse-to-elephant" curve exemplified by the fact that a mouse has an elevated RHR (nearly 500 bpm) compared to the elephant (nearly 30 bpm), while their respective lifespan is inversely proportional to the RHR (average longevity of 3 years for a mouse versus 60 years for an elephant); the second observation is exemplified by athletically fit people who have a lower RHR and tend to live longer than sedentary people (Speakman, 2005). Similarly, the association between low RHR and longevity is found in other animals like the leatherback sea turtle (Dermochelys coriacea) which has the longest lifespan among animals (up to 150 years); interestingly, this kind of turtle can have a "physiologically" low RHR down to nearly 1 bpm (Southwood *et al.*, 1999). In summary, the "heartbeat" hypothesis correlates a lower RHR and a lower metabolic rate with a longer longevity, and this is explained by a lower oxidative stress with subsequent lower free radicals with are involved in DNA mutation and cells apoptosis, which are associated with premature ageing and occurrence of diseases like cancer, hypertension and atherosclerosis.

1.3   Heart Rate as Risk Factor for Coronary Artery Disease

Many epidemiological studies have consistently shown that iRHR is predictive of cardiovascular mortality, mainly from CAD, even after adjustment with other CAD risk factors, such as hypertension, smoking and dyslipidemia (Palatini, 2007; Dyer *et al.*, 1980). HR is a clinical parameter relatively easy to measure in daily medical practice, however, measurement should be standardized in order to avoid false negative or false positive values; the resting period before measurement, the posture during measurement, the surrounding environmental conditions, the accuracy of the methodology used and the definition of normal values of HR are issues to take into consideration. The classical value of 100 bpm above which the rhythm is considered "abnormal" is not quite convincing and suitable, especially in patients with CAD (Vogel *et al.*, 2004; Palatini *et al.*, 2006). The definition of iRHR is still difficult given the lack of universal value above which HR is considered increased, however, and according to the cornerstone study of patients with CAD (Fox *et al.*, 2008), a HR ≥70 bpm is considered as iRHR in patients with CAD and it predisposes to higher risk of major cardiac events.

Nowadays, patients with CAD still suffer from a relatively high rate of adverse events (refractory angina pectoris, myocardial infarction, heart failure, sudden cardiac death), despite "optimal" therapy and "optimal" secondary prevention. In view of that, identification of some "ignored" or "neglected" factor predisposing to adverse event is essential and we estimate that iRHR is a missing link that needs to be addressed in this context in order to improve outcomes of CAD.

1.4   Physiology of Heart Rate Value

Classical values of "normal" HR are set between 60 and 100 bpm, and when HR is below 60 bpm the rhythm is classified as bradycardia while HR above 100 bpm is classified as tachycardia. The heart rhythm is generated in the sinoatrial node (Keith and Flack node); (Silverman & Hollman, 2007). Anatomically, the sinus node is formed from central P cells (pacemaker cells) and peripheral T cells (transitional cells) that transmit the impulse from the P cells to the surrounding atrial tissue. The sinoatrial node is located in the high right atrium at the junction of the crista terminalis with the superior vena cava. Intrinsic HR is defined as the proper rate when the heart is devoid of the autonomic nervous system influence on the heart; this can be achieved by administering Atropine (0.04 mg/kg) and Propranolol (0.2 mg/kg) simultaneously, leading to pharmacological denervation of the sinus node within nearly 5 minutes and the resultant HR is the proper intrinsic rate that is theoretically equal to 117.2 – [0.53 x Age] (Monfredi, 2013).

HR is a very subtle cardiovascular parameter, it is influenced by variable processes comprising the intrinsic sinus node function, the cardiovascular afferent signals and the central influx from the brain; the potential presence of a predetermined RHR for every individual as a central setup point is not established. Cardiac output is equal to the product of the stroke volume and the HR, and the heart is considered the servant of the organism rather than the commander, meaning that the basic metabolic rate adjusts the cardiac output by modulating the stroke volume and the HR; also this process requires the intervention of many actors, mainly the autonomic nervous system, baroreceptors, endothelial function, systolic and diastolic function, etc. (Monfredi *et al.*, 2013).

The cardiovascular regulation center which is located in the medulla integrates peripheral sensory data (afferent cardiovascular system inputs) with influx from higher brain centers, mainly from the hypothalamus. The hypothalamus amends the activity of the medullary centers in order to regulate the cardiovascular responses to emotion and stress. The medulla is the primary site in the brain for regulating the autonomic nervous system outflow to the heart, namely the sympathetic nerve with its positive chronotropic effect and the parasympathetic nerve with its negative chronotropic effect (Shaffer *et al.*, 2014). Moreover, the autonomic nervous system has a circadian variability with a maximal tone of the parasympathetic nerve at night while the sympathetic nervous system has rather a higher tone during the day, also psychological and physical stresses yield a higher sympathetic tone with subsequent iRHR.

During exertion, there is a gradual increase in HR which is usually proportional to the load of exertion. The gradual increase in HR is named the positive chronotropic response of the heart and it is mainly dependent on the sinus node function and on the autonomic nervous system. The maximal HR (MHR) is theoretically equal to [220–age] and the chronotropic reserve is defined as the MHR minus the RHR. The HR value during exertion basically is dependent on the factors that control the RHR, but also on physical fitness, exercise load, functional capacity, and maximal oxygen consumption capacity (VO2max) (Monfredi *et al.*, 2013).

1.5   Physiopathology of Heart Rate Value

Though "normal" rates are classically set as being within the range of 60 to 100 bpm, we estimate that this classification does not reflect the real physiology and pathology of RHR (Palatini, 1999). For instance, many subjects have a RHR between 50 and 60, they are asymptomatic and manage to have a normal life during all daily physiological conditions; in this context, when a subject has a RHR in this range while keeping an adapted chronotropic response up to the MHR, there are no sufficient arguments or definite criteria to consider such HR value as "abnormal" RHR or "bradycardia". To the best of our knowledge, and except for the documented cases of sinus node dysfunction, RHR slower than 60 bpm does not adversely affect morbidity or mortality.

Similarly, patients with iRHR (i.e. RHR 70–100) are classically considered having a "normal" RHR: however, multiple recent and semi recent trial (Tardif, 2009; Wang *et al.*, 2014) showed that iRHR even below 100 bpm is associated with adverse cardiovascular outcome, whether in healthy subjects or in patients with CAD; accordingly, we estimate that the upper limit of abnormal HR needs probably to be redefined (Palatini, 1999). In this chapter, we will discuss the case of iRHR in cases where no dysrhythmias or any extracardiac condition is documented as predisposing or causing iRHR or tachycardia; herein, we exclude cases of atrial fibrillation or other persistent supraventricular tachycardia, postural orthostatic tachycardia and inappropriate sinus tachycardia, also we exclude any extracardiac condition like organic dysautonomia or hyperthyroidism.

When addressing HR value, it is essential to differentiate between iRHR in healthy subjects and in patients with already documented cardiac conditions like heart failure, CAD or hypertension. In the former scenario, the discussion aims to show the independent causal association between iRHR and the subsequent occurrence of cardiovascular adverse events, in which case the iRHR is identified as a risk factor for cardiovascular morbidity. In the second scenario where iRHR is associated with cardiovascular conditions, iRHR may be a consequence of the condition itself (i.e. heart failure with consecutive tachycardia, etc), a direct causal factor (i.e. hypertension with iRHR correlated to increased sympathetic tone) or even a bystander phenomenon which is neither causal nor consecutive of the condition.

In all cases, we estimate that iRHR whether documented in healthy subjects or in patients with cardiac conditions is a marker of adverse cardiovascular events. In the following section, we will present and discuss the significance of HR in the pathogenesis of CAD with the perspective of a better management and prevention. Topics discussed relate to HR and atherosclerosis, criteria of HR normality, HR and hypertension, HR and endothelial dysfunction, HR and autonomic nervous system and inflammation, HR and diastolic dysfunction, HR in acute and chronic coronary syndrome, and the main trials studying HR in CAD.

2   Physiopathology of Resting Heart Rate, Interaction with Coronary Artery Disease and Associated Comorbidities

2.1   Heart Rate and Atherosclerosis

Heart rhythm is generated in the sinoatrial node which is located at the upper lateral segment of the right atrium; the sinoatrial node is irrigated by sinus node artery which is a branch of the right coronary artery, also the node is innervated by the autonomic nervous system which has a considerable control on HR. In this view, patients with CAD, namely when involving the right coronary artery, may exhibit a low RHR directly correlated to the poor sinus node irrigation with subsequent slow firing rate of the "physiological pacemaker" (Zahedi et al., 1999).

Atherosclerosis is derived from the Greek "athero", meaning wax referring to the central core of the plaque, and "sclerosis" meaning induration referring to the fibrous cap of the plaque. Processes involved in atherosclerosis include endothelial injury and dysfunction, intimal inflammation, lipid accumulation, smooth muscle cells proliferation and plaque formation. With continued local lipid accumulation, local inflammation and oxidative stress, atherosclerotic plaques exhibit remodeling over time and may evolve to high-risk plaques, which may rupture leading to matrix breakdown and atherothrombosis. Atherosclerosis occurs roughly in all arteries, and it is more common at branch points where shear stress is higher, also it has specific clinical manifestations in coronary arteries, namely angina and myocardial infarction.

Atherosclerosis is the main etiological factor leading to CAD, and conventional risk factors for developing CAD include dyslipidemia, hypertension, tobacco smoking and diabetes mellitus; other risk factors include obesity, sedentarity, family history, metabolic syndrome, type A personality and mental stress, older age, high C-reactive protein (CRP), chronic inflammation and increased homocysteine. Patients documented with atherosclerotic CAD associated with coronary calcification are at higher risk of cardiac events; coronary arterial calcium score- as assessed by cardiac computed tomography angiography, portends a higher lifetime coronary risk according to the Framingham risk score (Hulten et al., 2014).

The 2013 ESC guidelines reported that iRHR is a strong independent risk factor for adverse outcome in patients with stable CAD, with a linear relationship between RHR and major cardiovascular events; in this regard, the authors stated that HR reduction targeting a RHR below 60 bpm should be an important goal in the treatment of stable CAD (Montalescot et al., 2013).

CRP is a protein correlated with systemic inflammation, which is the body's response to injury or infection. The atherosclerotic process which contributes to the growth of arterial plaque and atherothrombosis reflects an endothelial injury and is associated with an increase in CRP. The 2012 ACCF/AHA guidelines for assessment of cardiovascular risk in asymptomatic adults state that measurement of CRP can be useful in selecting patients for statin therapy and is reasonable for cardiovascular risk assessment (Fihn *et al.*, 2012).

iRHR is proven to be an independent risk factor for atherosclerosis (Palatini, 1999), this risk remains highly significant after controlling for major risk factors of atherosclerosis suggesting that iRHR plays a direct role in the induction and progression of atherosclerosis; in this regard, iRHR has a direct action on the vascular risk induction, it is correlated to the increase in the frequency of the pulsatile arterial waves and therefore it increases arterial wall shear stress (Palatini & Julius, 2004; Palatini & Julius, 1999; Wang *et al.*, 2014). Moreover, oxidative stress, endothelial dysfunction and inflammation are crucial parameters to take into consideration when addressing prevention and management of CAD (da Cunha *et al.*, 2014).

2.2   Criteria for Assessment of Heart Rate and Indices of Normality

The values of RHR are different from one subject to another, and many factors are involved in the "setup" value of each individual. The potential existence of a central "setup" point that regulates HR value in each individual is not quite established. Emotional factors interfere with RHR via the neurohumoral axis, namely the autonomic nervous system and related hormones. On the other hand, many peripheral factors (cardiac output, body weight, lean mass, physical fitness, endothelial function, baroreceptors, ...) interact together to yield a RHR which is specific to each subject. Classically, HR above 100 bpm is considered abnormal and the subject is described as having tachycardia; however, such value of 100 bpm is not the gold standard criteria above which a HR value is considered abnormal (Vogel *et al.*, 2004; Palatini, 1999), and there are multiple studies reporting that HR value ≥70 bpm is considered abnormal given that it portends higher cardiovascular morbidity and mortality, both in normal subjects and in patients with CAD (Wang *et al.*, 2014; Palatini , 2006).

The conditions under which HR is measured are crucial and somewhat similar to those implemented for measurement of blood pressure. Five conditions are considered as significantly influential and must be met in order to yield a standard measurement of HR: (i) a resting period before measurement (i.e.; 5 minutes); (ii) the posture of the patient during measurement (i.e.; sitting position); (iii) environmental conditions such as surrounding temperature, visual and acoustic stimuli; (iv) method used to record HR value; and (v) data analysis, i.e., determination of normality, the normal value above which the subject is considered having iRHR. In most of the studies addressing RHR, such informations are almost completely lacking (Vogel *et al.*, 2004), and therefore we estimate that such a crucial parameter is not assessed objectively in many studies. In this regard, it is recommended to standardize HR measurements and more importantly to redefine normality. In this chapter, and according to the reviewed data, patients with HR value≥ 70 bpm were considered having iRHR (Fox *et al*, 2008; Palatini, 1999; Palatini, 2006) .

2.3   Heart Rate and Hypertension

Many studies have already shown that iRHR is associated with atherosclerosis, hypertension and adverse cardiovascular events (Palatini & Julius, 2004; Giannoglou *et al.*, 2008); furthermore, subjects with iRHR often exhibit metabolic disturbances such as insulin resistance, overweight, dyslipidemia and higher hematocrit (Palatini & Julius, 1999). Of note, sympathetic overactivity seems to be involved in both the iRHR and hypertension; iRHR may reflect the increased sympathetic tone, and in such case it is often associated with hypertension. However, hypertension in such cases can not be explained only by a direct effect of the iRHR, it is also related to the increase in peripheral vascular resistance and to the increased volemia. Moreover, iRHR and hypertension are often co-existent with endothelial dysfunction which may be a consequence or even causal of the two conditions (iRHR and hypertension) (Palatini & Julius, 1999).

2.4   Heart Rate and Endothelial Dysfunction

The correlation between RHR and endothelial function/dysfunction has not been extensively studied and many cardiovascular risk factors are known to have an adverse impact on the endothelial function, including hypertension, dyslipidemia, and diabetes. Endothelial function is a crucial parameter in the regulation of cardiovascular homeostasis, including HR, vasoactivity, preload, afterload, and cardiac output. Moreover, cardiac output is a direct result of the HR and stroke volume product. It is already established that the performance of structured physical activity improves the antioxidant capacity, decreases RHR and reduces oxidative stress, also it improves endothelial function as demonstrated by small artery reactive hyperaemia index (Merino *et al.*, 2015). The decrease in RHR in physically fit subjects is correlated to enhanced vagal tone, along with a better endothelial-mediated vasodilatation, and higher stroke volume at rest. Of note, the decrease in RHR in this context is in part involved in improving the endothelial function (decrease of mechanical shear stress).

It is already demonstrated that dyslipidemia exposes to oxidative stress and this condition impairs the endothelium-dependent relaxation which is mediated by nitric oxide (NO). The lack in NO in this context is due to the decreased endothelial NO synthase activity, increased NO inactivation and increased production of the endothelium-derived constricting factors (thromboxane A2, endothelin-1); in addition, the whole process is accompanied by local endothelial inflammation with an increase in CRP (Hayakawa & Raij, 1999).

Endothelial microparticles are complex vesicular structures that originate from activated endothelial cells, and they reflect pathological processes such as endothelial dysfunction, systemic inflammation, enhanced coagulation, and angiogenesis. Circulating endothelial microparticles are specifically increased in patients with CAD and their elevation is considered a biomarker of vascular damage. The baroreflex function is closely correlated to the endothelium, its function is mainly involved in blood pressure regulation via HR regulation and vasomotion modulation and this action is mediated via the autonomic nervous system. Any defect in the baroreflex function, whether related to endothelial or autonomic dysfunction, may lead to a decrease or increase in RHR;

in the latter case, the condition may lead to intermittent or persistent iRHR. (Ramchandra *et al.*, 2014)

iRHR is associated with increased systemic inflammation, oxidative stress and endothelial dysfunction; this phenomenon is likely to contribute to, though it does not fully explain, the increased morbidity and mortality in patients with iRHR (Nanchen *et al*, 2013). Of note, oxidative stress, endothelial dysfunction and increased CRP are involved in the pathogenesis of CAD, and accordingly, primary and secondary prevention of CAD must be based on correction of these physiopathological factors along with HRC. Endothelial dysfunction plays an important role in the development of atherosclerosis, also it predicts adverse cardiovascular outcomes independently of conventional cardiovascular risk factors. There have been tremendous improvements recently in CAD prevention and management, and such improvements are mainly focused on endothelial function. Atherosclerotic CAD should be managed on the basis of identifying and controlling not only traditional risk factors, but also non-traditional factors such as iRHR. Endothelial function represents an integrated index of all atherogenic and atheroprotective factors present in an individual including non-traditional factors, also it has a pivotal role in all phases of atherosclerosis, from initiation to atherothrombotic complications. (Thorin & Thorin-Trescases, 2009)

2.5   Heart Rate, Autonomic Nervous System and Inflammation

The increase in hs-CRP reflects an inflammatory process and it is often correlated with unbalanced cardiac autonomic function with subsequent increase in RHR; an independent association exists between inflammation and reduced vagal tone, and this phenomenon is mediated through several peripheral or central mechanisms that regulate immune and autonomic function (Nolan *et al.*, 2007). Markers of inflammation, such as CRP, IL-1b, IL-6, can influence the autonomic regulation of cardiovascular function through humoral and neural responses that affect local and systemic availability of glucocorticoids and catecholamines. Animal models have demonstrated that systemic administration of IL-1b increased the number of Fos-positive catecholamine cells in regions of the medulla that control the sympathetic outflow to the heart (A1 and C1 noradrenergic cells; C1 and C2 adrenergic cells) (Buller *et al*, 2003). In view of that, systemic inflammation is thought to yield an iRHR which is consecutive to the hypersympathetic tone and to the inflammatory cytokines released in the blood.

iRHR reflects increased sympathetic tone, also it is associated with impairment of HR variability and HR turbulence, and these two parameters are typically impaired post myocardial infarction. In addition, abnormal HR recovery reflects unbalanced cardiac autonomic function with a shift for a sympathetic overdrive; this phenomenon is commonly observed in subject with physical unfitness with subsequent iRHR. Abnormal HR recovery at one minute (defined as a decrease of HR less than 21 bpm the first minute after a "maximal" exercise) was associated with higher prevalence of CAD, predicting the presence but not the severity of CAD (Akyüz *et al*, 2014).

Increased sympathetic and decreased parasympathetic activities are associated with an increased risk of ventricular arrhythmias and sudden cardiac death; of note, such autonomic dysfunction is often associated with a decreased heart rate variability. In this context, the decreased heart rate variability is associated with an increased RHR, predicting cardiovascular and all-cause and mortality namely in patients with CAD (Pradhapan *et al*, 2014).

2.6   Heart Rate and Diastolic Dysfunction

The relationship between HR and diastolic function is already established, a persistent increase in RHR compromises diastolic filling, also it shortens diastole, the phase of cardiac cycle during which coronary circulation is taking place (Kneffel *et al.*, 2011). Moreover, cardiac output is the direct product of stroke volume and HR; stroke volume is directly dependent on systolic and diastolic function and any impairment in any of these is compensated by an increase in RHR in order to preserve cardiac output. In other words, diastolic dysfunction leads to iRHR and the reverse is true, iRHR shortens diastole and impairs diastolic function.

Coronary flow reserve is typically above 2.5 (compared to the baseline flow) in normal subjects, however it decreases significantly in patients with iRHR; arterial hypertension is a major etiologic factor of diastolic dysfunction and coronary flow reserve commonly decreases below 2.5 in hypertensive patients with diastolic dysfunction. In such cases, even patients who are free of intrinsic CAD may manifest exertional angina related to a decrease in coronary flow reserve. Of note, the independent association between the decrease in coronary flow reserve and diastolic dysfunction is encountered whatever is the origin of diastolic dysfunction, and HRC in such cases is of utmost importance in order to control symptoms, beyond classical anti-anginal therapy (Karayannis *et al.*, 2011).

Coronary flow occurs mainly during diastole and it is correlated to many factors including the duration of diastole, the aortic diastolic pressure and the coronary anatomy and function; the "suction-like" property of the coronary arteries during diastole is related to their vasoactive property which is correlated to the endothelial function and to the vascular wall structure; moreover, coronary perfusion is taking place mainly during diastole by an auxiliary pump, which is an elastic reservoir consisting of the aorta; in case of arterial calcification, the aorta becomes rigid and gradually becomes unable of generating sufficient pressure for adequate coronary perfusion and this is an example of diastolic dysfunction at the level of the vasculature that negatively affects coronary flow.

2.7   Heart Rate in Acute Coronary Syndrome

At the initial phase of acute coronary syndrome, patients presenting with iRHR are at higher risk of adverse cardiovascular outcome; patients with iRHR ≥90 bpm have the worse prognosis in this context (Asaad *et al.*, 2014). In the multicenter Canadian ACS Registries (Segev *et al.*, 2006), iRHR documented on admission of patients with ACS was found associated with a more advanced Killip grade and the concerned patients had an adverse prognostic outcome. Moreover, persistent iRHR after admission and during hospital stay reflects hemodynamic instability and is considered an independent predictor of increased in-hospital and 1-year death.

Similarly, HR at discharge has a major impact on long term prognosis following percutaneous coronary intervention in acute coronary syndromes (Jensen *et al.*, 2013): in this study, discharge HR was determined from a resting ECG, and iRHR was considered present when RHR was ≥ 60 bpm; outcomes were evaluated for all-cause mortality, cardiovascular death and non-fatal myocardial infarction during a follow-up period from 7 days to 2 years. Interestingly, iRHR was found significantly associated with all-cause mortality when compared to a reference group with RHR < 60 bpm [adjusted hazard ratios (95% CI): 4.5 for 60–69 bpm, 3.8 for 70–79 bpm, 4.3 for 80–89 bpm, and 16.9 for > 90 bpm]. Moreover, cardiovascular death/myocardial infarction was associated with a hazard ratio of 6.2 in patients with a discharge HR > 90 bpm compared to those with HR < 60 bpm and the authors concluded that revascularized patients with PCI for acute coronary syndrome have a poor prognosis when discharge RHR is elevated as defined in the study (> 60 bpm).

Fácila *et al* reported that a RHR ≥ 70 bpm after an acute coronary syndrome identifies a population that is at high risk of major cardiovascular events and higher mortality during follow-up; the authors suggested that an aggressive treatment in such patients must be implemented in order to achieve a RHR below 70 bpm which could translate into a better prognosis (Fácila, 2012).

2.8   Heart Rate and Coronary Microcirculation

Patients with microvascular angina usually do not respond adequately to classical anti-anginal therapy such as nitrates or beta-blockers; also management of microvascular angina is often empiric and this is related to the poor understanding of the pathophysiologic mechanisms and the possible heterogeneous nature of the disease. Despite optimal conventional anti-ischemic therapy, many patients still symptomatic and require additional therapeutic approach, also such patients often exhibit stable angina and have positive stress test despite a normal coronary angiogram; however, their coronary flow reserve is decreased. Patients in whom symptoms are inadequately controlled by standard anti-ischemic therapy respond well to rate control medication; in this regard, Ivabradine, an I(f) current inhibitor drug, has proven its efficacy in microvascular angina in combination with conventional anti-ischemic therapy (Meinertz *et al.*, 2011). Symptomatic improvement with Ivabradine is related to a decrease in RHR along with an improvement in HR profile during exercise; in addition, Ivabradine improves coronary flow reserve significantly, through HR reduction and by improving microvascular circulation (Skalidis *et al*, 2011).

2.9   Heart Rate Reduction Associated with the Development of Coronary Collaterals

Bradycardia has been shown to be associated with the development of collateral circulation in patients with CAD, this arteriogenic effect is due to the tangential fluid shear force at the endothelial cell layer during prolonged diastole (Patel *et al.*,2000) . In animal studies, it has been demonstrated that tangential fluid shear stress is a major trigger of collateral vascular growth (arteriogenesis); experimental lower-leg external counterpulsation triggered during diastole induces tangential endothelial shear stress, and such stress has been shown to effectively increase collateral circulation (Gloekler *et al*, 2010). Regular exercise training leads to a lower RHR, and the main beneficial effect of exercise could be the extension of diastole with prolonged action of the tangential shear force on the endothelium triggering coronary arteriogenic process (Vogel *et al.*, 2010). Tangential shear force τ (in dyne/cm²) is the product of blood viscosity and shear rate, which is the spatial rate of velocity change between different fluid layers adjacent to the endothelium and the endothelium itself. In view of this, a bradycardia-inducing drug that prolongs the diastolic time of the tangential shear force has theoretically a positive effect on collateral circulation development (Gloekler *et al.*, 2014).

2.10   Heart Rate in Patients with Stable Coronary Artery Disease (Chronic Coronary Syndrome)

2.10.1   Physiopathology of Coronary Artery Disease in Patients with iRHR

iRHR is an important pathophysiological variable that increases myocardial oxygen demand, it also limits tissue perfusion by reducing the duration of diastole, during which most myocardial perfusion occurs (Tardif *et al.*, 2009). Whether iRHR is a consequence or simply a marker of some comorbidities is not quite established; for instance, iRHR is encountered in endothelial dysfunction and oxidative stress, and both conditions predispose to CAD (Palatini & Julius, 2004). Multiple scenario are to be considered in such cases, iRHR could be causal, or a consequence of CAD (or a consequence of the relevant comorbidity, such as oxidative stress…); less likely, iRHR is an innocent bystander (epiphenomenon). In fact, these scenario are interdependent with some potential "complicity" in between, which means one factor may enhance or mask another one: for instance, iRHR predisposes to endothelial dysfunction, oxidative stress, and CAD and the reverse is true, both oxidative stress and endothelial dysfunction lead to iRHR causing a vicious circle in this context (Celik A *et al.*, 2012; Giannoglou *et al.*, 2008) . In view of this, we consider that iRHR is commonly encountered in CAD and associated comorbidities, whether as a causal factor, as a consequence or as an epiphenomenon; whatsoever is the scenario, we estimate that iRHR is a precious marker in CAD, with a potential value somewhat "similar" to that of hs-CRP, and accordingly, it may be implemented in this regard for risk assessment and for targeting therapy (Brito Díaz *et al.*, 2014).

Several epidemiological studies have reported that iRHR is associated with coronary atherosclerosis independently of other risk factors; the pathophysiologic mechanisms involved in the pro-atherosclerotic effect of iRHR are in part associated with the increased sympathetic tone and its deleterious effect (Giannoglou *et al.*, 2008). Moreover, iRHR increases the frequency of the tensile stress imposed on the arterial wall and prolongs the exposure of the coronary endothelium to the oscillatory shear stress; furthermore, iRHR increases the pulsatile motion of the heart and, therefore, the frequency of the periodically changing geometry of the coronary arteries, thereby affecting the local hemodynamic environment and local oscillatory shear stress. All these processes induce structural and functional changes at the level of the coronary endothelial cells, with a cumulative effect over time promoting atherosclerosis.

The pulsatile nature of the blood flow constitutes the major generator of the oscillatory shear stress, and HR determines directly the frequency of flow pulsation; therefore, its reduction could potentially decelerate the progression of atherosclerosis by alleviating the local atherogenic oscillatory shear stress (Chatzizisis & Giannoglou, 2006). Moreover, the coronary tree is exposed to the atherogenic effect of systemic risk factors, also endothelial gene expression through complex transduction processes intervene; in this process, each plaque exhibits an individual natural history of progression, regression, or stabilization, which is dependent on both systemic and local factors. Though the pathophysiologic mechanisms involved in the formation and remodeling of the atherosclerotic plaque are incompletely understood, decreasing RHR is of utmost importance to minimize the dynamic interplay between local shear stress, biology (molecular and cellular) of the vascular wall and systemic factors (inflammation, hypertension…) (Chatzizisis *et al.*, 2007).

2.10.2   Physiopathology of iRHR in Patients with Coronary Artery Disease and Other Comorbidities

High levels of sympathetic drive is documented in several cardiovascular diseases including postmyocardial infarction, chronic congestive heart failure and hypertension; the sympathetic overdrive is mediated through dysregulation of the afferent input along with a central dysregulation of autonomic balance. In CAD, the persistent or intermittent local myocardial ischemia generates afferent sympathetic input leading to hypersympathetic tone (Wang *et al.*, 2013 & Brito Díaz, 2014). Moreover, a significant component of sympathetic hyperactivity resides peripherally at the level of the postganglionic neuron, with increased release and impaired reuptake of norepinephrine in neurons of the satellite ganglia leading to a significant increase in RHR. Furthermore, sympathetic nerve sprouting after myocardial infarction is associated with NF-κB activation and this may be one additional mechanism responsible for iRHR. Such phenomena lead to higher myocardial oxygen demand, lower coronary reserve flow, also it may lead to a decrease in arrhythmia threshold, and coronary microvascular angiopathy (Shanks & Herring, 2013).

In patients with previous myocardial infarction, a local or diffuse myocardial dysfunction is a direct trigger of sympathetic overdrive with subsequent iRHR as a compensatory mechanism of the hemodynamic dysfunction; the size of the necrotic area is a main determinant of the hemodynamic dysfunction in this context. Hence, in order to improve outcome in myocardial infarction, it is essential to reduce infarct size which is influenced by the duration of coronary occlusion and the lack of collateral blood supply to the ischaemic zone. CAD is commonly associated with systolic and diastolic dysfunction, leading respectively to a decrease in stroke volume and preload. Given that HR is a major determinant of cardiac output, any decrease in the stroke volume or in the pre-load may generate a reflex tachycardia (increase in RHR) in order to compensate for the decrease in cardiac output.

2.11   Management of Coronary Artery Disease, the Role of RHR and Physical Activity

Cardiovascular diseases are the leading cause of death worldwide and CAD is the most prevalent and most preventable form of cardiovascular diseases. The control of risk fac-tors is essential in this regard whether via primary or secondary prevention. Modifiable risk factors include mainly dyslipidemia, smoking, hypertension, diabetes mellitus, obe-sity and sedentary lifestyle, also other risk factors control comprises prevention and management of endothelial dysfunction, chronic inflammation, oxidative stress and CRP increase. Management of CAD comprises primarily medical therapy, percutaneous coronary intervention and coronary artery bypass grafts.

iRHR is an emergent risk factor of CAD, however it is not currently considered as one of the conventional modifiable risk factors of cardiovascular diseases, though HR assessment and HRC is probably – among other CAD risk factors- the most "easy and accessible" factor to assess and to manage, whether through medication and/or through lifestyle modification. HRC aims to control and lower iRHR, by controlling potential causal factors for iRHR like overweight, also by lifestyle changes like regular physical exercise to acquire physical fitness, or by medications like I(f) current inhibitor drug (Ivabradine). Many pharmacological agents are useful for HRC, and they are qualified as negative chronotropic drugs such as non-dihydropyridine calcium channel blockers and β-blockers. However, these agents are not primarily targeting HR, their effect is multifaceted comprising vasoactive effect, inotropic effect, along with modulation of the diastolic function, the electrophysiological excitability and conductivity.

Agents that are purely targeting the sinoatrial node have been described first in 1994, these agents (S-16257 and UL-FS 49) were tested on rabbit and guinea-pig cardiac preparations (Thollon *et al.*, 1994) . The S-16257, was first tested on humans in 1998 (Ragueneau *et al.*, 1998) under the brand name "Ivabradine"; it was tested on healthy volunteers as a new bradycardic agent with a direct effect on the sinus node, also its N-dealkylated metabolite, S-18982, has shown a bradycardic activity. Interestingly, the effects of Ivabradine on HR were studied at rest and during exercise tests, and both the parental compound and its metabolite, the S-18982 showed a decrease in HR whether at rest or during exercise. A pharmacokinetic and pharmacodynamic analysis showed that S-18982 is responsible for the initial bradycardic effect, whereas the parent compound is responsible for the duration of action.

Cardiac rehabilitation is a recognized procedure for promoting physical fitness, increasing maximal oxygen consumption and improving endothelial function; moreo-ver, one of the major benefit of cardiac rehabilitation is mediated through decreasing RHR, whether implemented as primary prevention or as secondary prevention (Merino *et al.*, 2015). Outside a structured cardiac rehabilitation program, the role of physical activity is also beneficial; however, the "amount" of such physical activity (i.e.; intensity, duration and frequency) and the type (i.e.; isotonic versus isometric) is essential in this context and has to be adapted to the subject condition.

A recent meta-analysis (Sattelmair *et al.*, 2011) showed that "some physical activity is better than none" and "additional benefits occur with more physical activity." Of note, the entire process through which physical activity lowers cardiovascular morbidity and mortality is not fully elucidated, however, it is established that chronic and regular physical activity decreases RHR, and improves both endothelial function and functional capacity. Obesity by itself predisposes to iRHR and to sinus tachycardia, and this is a "physiological" response of the heart to the increased body mass index with subsequent increase in metabolic rate; Interestingly, Shigetoh (Shigetoh *et al.*, 2009) reported that iRHR may predispose to the development of obesity and diabetes mellitus, suggesting that the sympathetic nervous system may play a role in this context. Metabolic syndrome is characterized by various metabolic abnormalities in an individual along with an increased risk for the development of type 2 diabetes and cardiovascular diseases. Metabolic syndrome is a relatively frequent syndrome with a prevalence in the general population of approximately 25%; of note, central fat accumulation and insulin resistance are common denominators encountered in metabolic syndrome. Subjects with metabolic syndrome have a predominance of the sympathetic nervous system and the mechanisms linking metabolic syndrome with sympathetic activation are complex and not clearly understood; whether sympathetic overactivity is involved in the development of the metabolic syndrome or is a consequence of it remains to be elucidated. Whatsoever is the scenario, sympathetic nervous system activation leads to iRHR, and a decrease in HR variability. The augmented sympathetic activity in individuals with metabolic syndrome worsens the prognosis of this high-risk population, however, intervention studies have demonstrated that autonomic disturbances in metabolic syndrome are reversible and iRHR can be managed with weight control and lifestyle changes (Tentolouris *et al.*, 2008).

2.12   Main Studies in RHR, Role of I(f) Current Inhibitor Drug (Ivabradine) in Coronary Artery Disease

Borer *et al.*, 2003;(n = 360); randomized, double-blind, placebo-controlled, multicentre study in patients with stable CAD and chronic stable angina; patients were randomly assigned to receive Ivabradine or placebo. Ivabradine produced dose-dependent improvement in exercise tolerance and time to development of ischemia during exercise and the authors concluded that Ivabradine is effective and safe in stable CAD (Borer *et al*, 2003).

Ruzyllo *et al.*, 2007; (n = 1195); randomized, double-blind, parallel-group, multicentre study; comparison of the antianginal and anti-ischaemic effects of Ivabradine with the calcium channel antagonist amlodipine. In patients with stable angina, Ivabradine has comparable efficacy to amlodipine in improving exercise tolerance, a superior effect on the reduction of rate-pressure product (a surrogate marker of myocardial oxygen consumption) and similar safety (Ruzyllo *et al.*, 2007).

BEAUTIFUL study, 2008; (n = 12473); The landmark study addressing RHR and CAD is the BEAUTIFUL study (*Evaluation of the* I(f) *inhibitor ivabradine in patients with coronary disease and left ventricular dysfunction*); multicentric, randomized, international, double-blind placebo-controlled study designed to evaluate the superiority of Ivabradine over placebo in reducing cardiovascular events in patients with stable CAD and left ventricular systolic dysfunction (ejection fraction < or = 39%). The study results showed that RHR ≥70 bpm is a marker for subsequent cardiovascular death and morbidity. Though Ivabradine treatment does not affect the primary composite outcome (cardiovascular death, or admission to hospital for new-onset or worsening heart failure) in patients with HR ≥70 bpm, it reduced admission to hospital for fatal and non-fatal myocardial infarction, also it reduced the need for coronary revascularisation. Accordingly, the authors concluded that Ivabradine is useful to reduce the incidence of CAD adverse outcomes in the subgroup of patients with RHR ≥70 bpm (Fox *et al.*, 2008).

ASSOCIATE, 2009; (n = 889); randomized, double-blind, placebo-controlled, multicentric study in patients with chronic stable angina; the study was designed to evaluate the anti-anginal and anti-ischaemic efficacy of the selective I(f) current inhibitor Ivabradine in patients with chronic stable angina pectoris receiving beta-blocker therapy. The combination was well tolerated (ivabradine 7.5 mg twice a day), only 1.1% of patients withdrew owing to sinus bradycardia. The authors concluded that the combination of Ivabradine and atenolol in clinical practice in patients with chronic stable angina pectoris produced additional efficacy with no untoward effect on safety or tolerability (Tardif *et al.*, 2009).

REDUCTION, 2009; (n = 4,954); multicentric, open-label, observational study in patients with stable angina pectoris. Patients with stable angina pectoris received Ivabradine and underwent a follow-up for 4 months. The HR, angina pectoris attacks, overall efficacy, and tolerance were evaluated. HR was reduced by 12.4 ± 12.2 bpm; Ivabradine is highly effective and well tolerated in the treatment of patients with symptomatic CAD (Köster *et al.*, 2009).

Tendera M *et al.*, 2009; (n = 2,425); pooled analysis of five randomized, double-blind, parallel-group in patients with angina pectoris, with a follow up of 4 months; Ivabradine was administered at a dosage of 5 to 10 mg, twice daily. Results: change in RHR: –14.5 %; change in the number of angina attacks per week: –59.4 % ; change in the consumption of nitrates: –53.7 %. Conclusion: the antianginal efficacy of Ivabradine was consistent across all the subpopulations analyzed, independent of the severity of angina and the presence of a comorbidity (Tendera *et al.* 2009).

Amosova *et al.*, 2011; (n = 29); randomized, parallel-group, single-blind study. Objective: to test the antianginal and anti-ischemic efficacy and hemodynamic profile of Ivabradine plus bisoprolol in patients with stable angina. Results: addition of Ivabradine improved exercise capacity, also chronotropic reserve significantly improved with Ivabradine. The authors concluded that combining Ivabradine with low dose bisoprolol in stable angina patients produces additional antianginal and anti-ischemic benefits and improves chronotropic reserve (Amosova *et al.*, 2011).

BEAUTIFUL Holter substudy, 2011; (n = 840); holter substudy of the BEAUTIFUL trial, duration 6 months. Ivabradine 5–7.5 mg bid vs placebo to test the efficacy on HR reduction over 24-hour. In Ivabradine group, waking vs sleeping HR reduction was 6.8 vs 5.2 bpm. More ivabradine patients than placebo patients had HR episodes < 50 bpm, but there was no between-group difference in episode severity (Tendera *et al.*, 2011).

BEAUTIFUL ECHO substudy, 2011; (*n* = 590); echocardiographic substudy of the BEAUTIFUL trial. Duration: 3–12 months. Ivabradine 5–7.5 mg bid vs placebo; the study evaluated the effects of HR reduction with Ivabradine on left ventricular size with a primary end-point the change in left ventricular end-systolic volume index and function and the cardiac biomarker N-terminal pro-brain natriuretic peptide (NT-proBNP). Results: treatment with Ivabradine was associated with a decrease in left ventricular end-systolic volume index, an increase in ejection fraction; the reduction in left ventricular end-systolic volume index was related to the degree of HR reduction with ivabradine. There were no differences in any other echocardiographic parameters or NT-proBNP. The authors concluded that Ivabradine may reverse detrimental left ventricular remodeling in patients with CAD and left ventricular systolic dysfunction (Ceconi *et al.*, 2011).

Riccioni G, 2013; substudy of ASSOCIATE trial. Ivabradine reduces the myocardial oxygen demand at rest and during exercise, it has no relevant negative effects on cardiac conduction, contractility, relaxation or repolarization; moreover, Ivabradine has no significant impact on systolic or diastolic blood pressure at rest or during exercise and reduces HR in all stages of physical exercise. Of note, these benefits are independent of baseline HR, confirming that HR reduction with Ivabradine is beneficial in all patients, even with β-blocker therapy, when RHR is above 60 bpm (Riccioni, 2013).

ADDITIONS, 2014; (*n* = 2330); multicentric, open-label, observational study in patients with stable angina pectoris. The study evaluated the efficacy, safety, and tolerability of Ivabradine added to β-blocker, and its effect on angina symptoms and quality of life. After 4 months of treatment with Ivabradine (mean dose 12.37 ± 2.95 mg/day), HR decreased by 19.4 ± 11.4 bpm. The authors concluded that addition of Ivabradine to β-blockers was effective in reducing HR, number of angina attacks, and nitrate consumption, also it improves the quality of life in patients with stable angina pectoris (Müller-Werdan *et al*, 2014).

3   Clinical Implications and Conclusion

iRHR is an independent risk factor for cardiovascular diseases, namely hypertension, heart failure and CAD. Many parameters intervene in the "setup" value of RHR in healthy subjects, and the potential presence of a central setup value is not quite established. Drugs reducing RHR (i.e. beta-blockers, Ivabradine) have the potential to improve cardiovascular outcome in patients with CAD, especially post coronary events. Interventions for reducing HR constitute a reasonable therapeutic goal in CAD, therefore prevention and management of CAD should take into consideration HR value, and a HR value < 70 bpm is currently the most valid and recognized value below which CAD risk is decreased (Brito Díaz *et al.*, 2014) .

Ivabradine is an I(f) current inhibitor that specifically lower RHR via direct action on sinoatrial node, without any direct effect on myocardial contractility, preload or afterload. Its beneficial effect extends beyond rate lowering (Riccioni, 2013), it has also a beneficial effect on collateral circulation (angiogenesis), it increases coronary flow reserve and by slowing HR, it has the property to decrease vascular shear stress and atherosclerotic process.

Lowering RHR may be achieved with physiological methods like regular physical exercise or cardiac rehabilitation. In this regard, physical activity, whether implemented as a primary process or as cardiac rehabilitation, should be targeting a RHR < 70 bpm mainly in patients with CAD. Physical exercise has the potency to improve microcirculation, to promote collateral circulation, also to decrease sympathetic overdrive which is involved in CAD pathophysiology.

β-blockers are established as gold-standard therapy post myocardial infarction, however patients with stable CAD and without prior myocardial infarction may benefit from the I(f) current inhibitor (Ivabradine) when RHR ≥70 bpm, as stand-alone therapy or in combination with β-blockers; however, in patients without CAD and with RHR above 70 bpm, primary prevention of CAD should mainly be implemented via structured physical exercise. Accordingly, HRC should be included in the armamentarium for fighting CAD as primary or as secondary prevention.

HR is an emergent cardiovascular risk factor and should be considered in every patient with CAD, since it is an easily measurable and a reproducible parameter; in this context, it can be viewed at as a second hs-CRP, a risk marker of cardiovascular diseases. With our current knowledge of the contribution of RHR to CAD, it is important to view this parameter from a comprehensive angle in order to prevent and improve outcomes in CAD: from endothelial dysfunction and oxidative stress to atherogenesis, researchers and clinicians must focus on the potential impact of any atherosclerotic condition or factor, including RHR in order to provide a tailored and individualized management.

References

Akyüz, A., Alpsoy, S., Akkoyun, D.C., et al. (2014). Heart rate recovery may predict the presence of coronary artery disease. Anadolu Kardiyol Derg ,14: 351–356.

Amosova, E., Andrejev, E., Zaderey, I. et al. (2011). Efficacy of ivabradine in combination with Beta-blocker versus uptitration of Beta-blocker in patients with stable angina. Cardiovasc Drugs Ther. , 25(6):531–537.

Asaad, N., El-Menyar, A., AlHabib, K.F., et al. (2014). Initial heart rate and cardiovascular outcomes in patients presenting with acute coronary syndrome. Acute Card Care., 16(2):49–56.

Borer, J.S., Fox, K., Jaillon, P. et al. (2003). Antianginal and antiischemic effects of ivabradine, an I(f) inhibitor, in stable angina: a randomized, double-blind, multicentered, placebo-controlled trial. Circulation. , 107(6):817–823.

Brito Díaz, B., Alemán Sánchez, J.J. & Cabrera de León, A. (2014). Resting heart rate and cardiovascular disease. Med Clin (Barc)., 143(1):34–38.

Buller, K.M., Dayas, C.V. & Day, T.A. (2003). Descending pathways from the paraventricular nucleus contribute to the recruitment of brainstem nuclei following a systemic immune challenge. Neuroscience. , 118(1):189–203.

Ceconi, C., Freedman, S.B., Tardif, J.C. et al. (2011). Effect of heart rate reduction by ivabradine on left ventricular remodeling in the echocardiographic substudy of BEAUTIFUL. Int J Cardiol. , 146(3):408–414.

Celik A, Koç F, Kadi H, et al. (2012). Inflammation is related to unbalanced cardiac autonomic functions in hypertension: an observational study. Anadolu Kardiyol Derg., 12(3):233–240.

Chatzizisis, Y.S. & Giannoglou, G.D. (2006). Pulsatile flow: a critical modulator of the natural history of atherosclerosis. Med Hypotheses., 67(2):338–340.

Chatzizisis, Y.S., Coskun, A.U., Jonas, M., et al. (2007). Role of endothelial shear stress in the natural history of coronary atherosclerosis and vascular remodeling: molecular, cellular, and vascular behavior. J Am Coll Cardiol. , 49(25):2379–2393.

da Cunha, N.V., Pinge-Filho, P., Panis, C., et al. (2014). Decreased endothelial nitric oxide, systemic oxidative stress, and increased sympathetic modulation contribute to hypertension in obese rats. Am J Physiol Heart Circ Physiol.,306(10):H1472–80.

Dyer, A.R., Persky, V., Stamler, J., et al. (1980). Heart rate as a prognostic factor for coronary heart disease and mortality: findings in three Chicago epidemiologic studies. Am J Epidemiol, 112: 736–749.

Fácila, L., Morillas, P., Quiles, J., et al. (2012). Prognostic significance of heart rate in hospitalized patients presenting with myocardial infarction. World J Cardiol., 4(1):15–9.

Fihn, S.D., Gardin, J.M., Abrams, J., et al. (2012). 2012 ACCF/AHA/ACP/AATS/PCNA/ SCAI/STS Guideline for the diagnosis and management of patients with stable ischemic heart disease: a report of the American College of Cardiology foundation/American Heart Association Task Force on Practice Guidelines, and the American College of Physicians, American Association for Thoracic Surgery, Preventive Cardiovascular Nurses Association, Society for Cardiovascular Angiography and Interventions, and Society of Thoracic Surgeons. J Am Coll Cardiol., 60(24):e44–e164.

Fox, K., Ford, I., Steg, P.G., Tendera, M., & Ferrari, R.(2008) ; BEAUTIFUL Investigators. Ivabradine for patients with stable coronary artery disease and left-ventricular systolic dysfunction (BEAUTIFUL): a randomised, double-blind, placebo-controlled trial. Lancet.,372 (9641):807–816.

Giannoglou, G.D., Chatzizisis, Y.S., Zamboulis, C., et al. (2008). Elevated heart rate and atherosclerosis: an overview of the pathogenetic mechanisms. Int J Cardiol. ,126(3):302–312.

Gloekler, S., Meier, P., de Marchi, S.F., et al. (2010). Coronary collateral growth by external counterpulsation: a randomised controlled trial. Heart., 96:202–207.

Gloekler, S., Traupe, T., Stoller,M. et al. (2014). The Effect of Heart Rate Reduction by Ivabradine on Collateral Function in Patients With Chronic Stable Coronary Artery Disease Heart. , 100(2):160–166.

Hayakawa, H., Raij, L. (1999). Relationship between hypercholesterolaemia, endothelial dysfunction and hypertension. J Hypertens., 17(5):611–619.

Hulten, E., Villines, T.C., Cheezum, M.K., et al. (2014). Calcium score, coronary artery disease extent and severity, and clinical outcomes among low Framingham risk patients with low vs high lifetime risk: results from the CONFIRM registry. J Nucl Cardiol. , 21(1):29–37

Jensen, M.T., Kaiser, C., Sandsten, K.E., et al. (2013). Heart rate at discharge and long-term prognosis following percutaneous coronary intervention in stable and acute coronary syndromes-results from the BASKET PROVE trial. Int J Cardiol., 168(4):3802–3806.

Kannel, W.B., Kannelm C., Paffenbarger, R.S.Jr & Cupples, L.A. (1987). Heart rate and cardiovascular mortality in the Framingham study. Am Heart J, 113:1489–1494.

Karayannis, G., Giamouzis, G., Alexandridis, E., et al. (2011). Prevalence of impaired coronary flow reserve and its association with left ventricular diastolic function in asymptomatic individuals with major cardiovascular risk factors. Eur J Cardiovasc Prev Rehabil., 18(2):326–333.

Kneffel, Z., Varga-Pintér, B., Tóth, M., et al. (2011). Relationship between the heart rate and E/A ratio in athletic and non-athletic males. Acta Physiol Hung., 98(3):284–93.

Köster, R., Kaehler, J. & Meinertz, T. (2009). Treatment of stable angina pectoris by ivabradine in every day practice: the REDUCTION study. Am Heart J., 158(4):e51–7.

Levine, H.J. (1997). Rest heart rate and life expectancy. J Am Coll Cardiol. ,30(4):1104–1106. Speakman, J.R. (2005). Body size, energy metabolism and lifespan. J Exp Biol., 208 (9):1717–1730.

Meinertz, T., Köster, R. (2011). New agents for the therapy of angina pectoris. Internist (Berl). ,52(7):894–6, 898–900.

Merino, J., Ferré, R., Girona, J., et al. (2015). Physical activity below the minimum international recommendations improves oxidative stress, ADMA levels, resting heart rate and small artery endothelial function. Clin Investig Arterioscler. , 27(1):9–16.

Monfredi, O., Maltsev, V.A. & Lakatta, E.G. (2013). Modern concepts concerning the origin of the heartbeat. Physiology (Bethesda)., 28(2):74–92.

Montalescot, G., Sechtem, U., Achenbach, S. et al. (2013). 2013 ESC guidelines on the management of stable coronary artery disease: the Task Force on the management of stable coronary artery disease of the European Society of Cardiology. Eur Heart J., 34(38):2949–3003.

Müller-Werdan, U., Stöckl, G., Ebelt, H. et al.(2014). Ivabradine in combination with beta-blocker reduces symptoms and improves quality of life in elderly patients with stable angina pectoris: Age-related results from the ADDITIONS study. Exp Gerontol. , 59C:34–41.

Nanchen, D., Stott, D.J., Gussekloo, J., et al. (2013). Resting heart rate and incident heart failure and cardiovascular mortality in older adults: role of inflammation and endothelial dysfunction: the PROSPER study. Eur J Heart Fail., 15(5):581–588.

Nolan, R.P., Reid, G.J., Seidelin, P.H., et al. (2007). C-reactive protein modulates vagal heart rate control in patients with coronary artery disease. Clin Sci (Lond)., 112(8):449–456.

Palatini, P. (1999). Heart rate as a risk factor for atherosclerosis and cardiovascular mortality: the effect of antihypertensive drugs. Drugs., 57(5):713–724.

Palatini, P. (1999). Need for a revision of the normal limits of resting heart rate. Hypertension. ,33(2):622–625.

Palatini, P. (2006). Heart rate: a cardiovascular risk factor that can no longer be ignored. G Ital Cardiol (Rome)., 7(2):119–128.

Palatini, P. (2007). Heart rate as an independent risk factor for cardiovascular disease: current evidence and basic mechanisms. Drugs, 67(2): 3–13.

Palatini, P. & Julius, S. (1999). The physiological determinants and risk correlations of elevated heart rate. Am J Hypertens.,12(1 Pt 2):3S–8S.

Palatini, P. & Julius, S. (2004). Elevated heart rate: a major risk factor for cardiovascular disease. Clin Exp Hypertens., 26(7–8):637–644.

Palatini, P., Benetos, A., Grassi, G., et al. (2006); European Society of Hypertension. Identification and management of the hypertensive patient with elevated heart rate: statement of a European Society of Hypertension Consensus Meeting. J Hypertens, 24: 603–610.

Patel, S., Breall, J., Diver, D., et al. (2000). Bradycardia is associated with development of coronary collateral vessels in humans. Coron Artery Dis., 11:467–472.

Pradhapan, P., Tarvainen, M.P., Nieminen, T. et al.(2014). Effect of heart rate correction on pre- and post-exercise heart rate variability to predict risk of mortality-an experimental study on the FINCAVAS cohort. Front Physiol., 5:208.

Ragueneau I, Laveille C, Jochemsen R, et al. (1998). Pharmacokinetic-pharmacodynamic modeling of the effects of ivabradine, a direct sinus node inhibitor, on heart rate in healthy volunteers. Clin Pharmacol Ther. , 64(2):192–203.

Ramchandra, R., Hood, S.G. & May, C.N. (2014). Central exogenous nitric oxide decreases cardiac sympathetic drive and improves baroreflex control of heart rate in ovine heart failure. Am J Physiol Regul Integr Comp Physiol., 307(3):R271–80.

Riccioni, G. (2013). The benefits of ivabradine are independent of resting heart rate. Future Cardiol., 9(3):313–315.

Ruzyllo, W., Tendera, M., Ford, I. et al. (2007). Antianginal efficacy and safety of ivabradine compared with amlodipine in patients with stable effort angina pectoris: a 3-month randomised, double-blind, multicentre, noninferiority trial. Drugs., 67(3):393–405.

Sattelmair, J., Pertman, J., Ding, E.L., et al. (2011). Dose response between physical activity and risk of coronary heart disease: a meta-analysis. Circulation. ,124(7):789–795.

Segev, A., Strauss, B.H., Tan, M., et al. (2006). Prognostic significance of admission heart failure in patients with non-ST-elevation acute coronary syndromes (from the Canadian Acute Coronary Syndrome Registries). Am J Cardiol. , 98(4):470–473.

Shaffer, F., McCraty, R. & Zerr, C.L. (2014). A healthy heart is not a metronome: an integrative review of the heart's anatomy and heart rate variability. Front Psychol.,5:1040.

Shanks, J. & Herring, N. (2013). Peripheral cardiac sympathetic hyperactivity in cardiovascular disease: role of neuropeptides. Am J Physiol Regul Integr Comp Physiol. , 305(12):R1411–20.

Shigetoh, Y., Adachi, H., Yamagishi, S., et al. (2009). Higher heart rate may predispose to obesity and diabetes mellitus: 20-year prospective study in a general population. Am J Hypertens. , 22(2):151–155.

Silverman, M.E. & Hollman, A.(2007). Discovery of the sinus node by Keith and Flack: on the centennial of their 1907 publication. Heart. ,93(10):1184–1187.

Skalidis, EI., Hamilos, M.I., Chlouverakis, G., et al. (2011). Ivabradine improves coronary flow reserve in patients with stable coronary artery disease. Atherosclerosis. , 215(1):160–165.

Southwood, A.L., Andrews, R.D., Lutcavage, M.E., et al. (1999). Heart rates and diving behavior of leatherback sea turtles in the eastern pacific ocean. J Exp Biol.,202 (9):1115–1125.

Speakman, J.R., Selman, C., McLaren, J.S. & Harper, E.J. (2002). Living Fast, Dying When? The Link between Aging and Energetics. J Nutr.,132(6):1583S–97S.

Stessman, J., Jacobs, J.M., Stessman-Lande, I., Gilon, D. & Leibowitz, D. (2013). Aging, resting pulse rate, and longevity. J Am Geriatr Soc. ,61(1):40–45.

Tardif, J.C. (2009). Heart rate as a treatable cardiovascular risk factor. Br Med Bull, 90:71–84.

Tardif, J.C., Ponikowski, P., Kahan, T. et al. (2009). Efficacy of the I(f) current inhibitor ivabradine in patients with chronic stable angina receiving beta-blocker therapy: a 4-month, randomized, placebo-controlled trial. Eur Heart J. , 30(5):540–548.

Tendera, M., Borer, J.S. & Tardif, J.C. (2009). Efficacy of I(f) inhibition with ivabradine in different subpopulations with stable angina pectoris. Cardiology. , 114(2):116–125.

Tendera, M., Talajic, M., Robertson, M., et al. (2011). Safety of ivabradine in patients with coronary artery disease and left ventricular systolic dysfunction (from the BEAUTIFUL Holter Substudy). Am J Cardiol. , 107(6):805–811.

Tentolouris, N., Argyrakopoulou, G. & Katsilambros, N. (2008). Perturbed autonomic nervous system function in metabolic syndrome. Neuromolecular Med., 10(3):169–178.

Thollon, C., Cambarrat, C., Vian, J. et al. (1994). Electrophysiological effects of S 16257, a novel sino-atrial node modulator, on rabbit and guinea-pig cardiac preparations: comparison with UL-FS 49. Br J Pharmacol., 112(1):37–42.

Thorin, E. & Thorin-Trescases, N. (2009). Vascular endothelial ageing, heartbeat after heartbeat. Cardiovasc Res., 84(1):24–32.

Vogel, C.U., Wolpert, C. & Wehling, M. (2004). How to measure heart rate? Eur J Clin Pharmacol., 60(7):461–466.

Vogel,R., Traupe, T., Steiger, V.S., et al. (2010). Physical coronary arteriogenesis: a human "model" of collateral growth promotion. Trends Cardiovasc Med, 20:129–133.

Wang, A., Chen, S., Wang, C., et al. (2014). Resting Heart Rate and Risk of Cardiovascular Diseases and All-Cause Death: The Kailuan Study PLoS One., 9(10):e110985.

Wang, Y., Suo, F. & Liu, J. (2013). Myocardial infarction induces sympathetic hyperinnervation via a nuclear factor-κB-dependent pathway in rabbit hearts. Neurosci Lett., 535:128–133.

Zahedi, A., Floras, J.S. & Burns, R.J. (1999). Absence of heart rate increase during inferoposterior left ventricular hypoperfusion caused by dipyridamole infusion. Can J Cardiol. , 15(12):1345–1349.

www.ingramcontent.com/pod-product-compliance
Lightning Source LLC
Chambersburg PA
CBHW061819210326
41599CB00034B/7050